The Complete Mediterranean Soups and Salads Cookbook

Don't miss incredibly delicious recipes to eat healthy and give your meals a boost.

Hanna Briggs

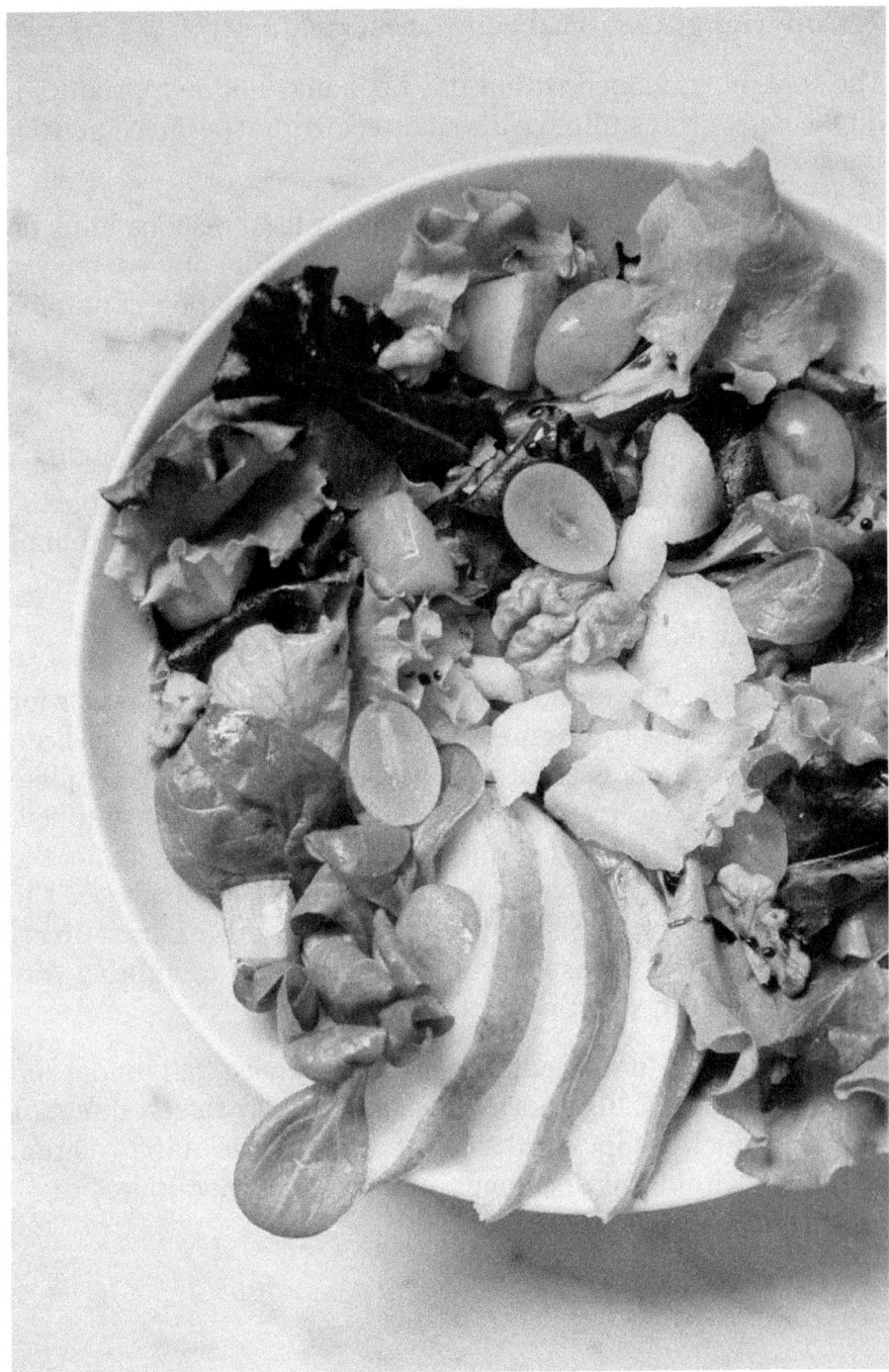

Table of contents

Introduction

Consuming the Mediterranean diet minimalizes the use of processed foods. It has been related to a reduced level of risk in developing numerous chronic diseases. It also enhances life expectancy. Several kinds of research have demonstrated many benefits in preventing cardiovascular disease, atrial fibrillation, breast cancer, and type 2 diabetes. Many pieces of evidence indicated a pattern that leads to low lipid, reduction in oxidative stress, platelet aggregation, and inflammation, and modification of growth factors and hormones involved in cancer.

Reduces Heart Diseases

According to research studies, the Mediterranean diet, which focuses on omega-3 ingredients and mono-saturated fats, reduces heart disease risk. It decreases the chances of cardiac death. The use of olive oil maintains the blood pressure levels. It is suitable for reducing hypertension. It also helps in combating the disease-promoting impacts of oxidation. This diet discourages the use of hydrogenated oils and saturated fats, which can cause heart disease.

Weight-loss

If you have been looking for diet plans for losing weight without feeling hungry, the Mediterranean diet can give you long term results. It is one of the best approaches. It is sustainable as it provides the most realistic approach to eat to feel full and energetic. This diet mostly consists of nutrient-dense food. It gives enough room for you to choose between low-carb and lower protein food. Olive oil consumed in this diet has antioxidants, natural vitamins, and some crucial fatty acids. It all improves your overall health. The Mediterranean diet focuses on natural foods, so there is very little room for junk and processed foods contributing to health-related issues and weight gain.

Most people trying the Mediterranean diet have gained positive results in cutting their weight. It is a useful option for someone looking forward to weight-loss as it provides the most unique and simple way to lose the overall calories without even changing your lifestyle that much. When you try to decrease calorie intake, losing weight is inevitable dramatically. But it will not benefit you. It will cause many health problems for you, including severe muscle loss. When you go for a Mediterranean diet, the body moves towards a sustainable model that burns calories slowly. So, it is crucial to practice the right approach and choose fat burning and more effective weight loss.

Prevents Cancer

The cornerstone of this diet is plant-based ingredients, especially vegetables and fruits. They help in preventing cancer. A plant-based diet provides antioxidants that help in protecting your DNA from damage and cell mutation. It also helps in lowering inflammation and delaying tumor growth. Various studies found that olive oil is a natural way to prevent cancer. It also decreases colon and bowel cancers. The plant-based diet balances blood sugar. It also sustains a healthy weight.

Prevents Diabetes

Numerous studies found that this healthy diet functions as an anti-inflammatory pattern, which helps fight the diseases related to chronic inflammation, Type 2 diabetes, and metabolic syndrome. It is considered very effective in preventing diabetes as it controls the insulin levels, which is a hormone to control the blood sugar levels and causes weight gain. Intake of a well-balanced diet consisting of fatty acids alongside some healthy carbohydrates and proteins is the best gift to your body. These foods help your body in burning fats more efficiently, which also provides energy. Due to the consumption of these kinds of foods, the insulin resistance level becomes non-existent, making it impossible to have high blood sugar.

Anti-aging

Choosing a Mediterranean diet without suffering from malnutrition is the most efficient and consistent anti-aging intervention. It undoubtedly expands lifespan, according to the research. The study found that the longevity biomarkers, i.e., body temperature and insulin level, and the DNA damage decreased significantly in humans by the Mediterranean diet. Other mechanisms also prove the claim made by researchers in explaining the anti-aging effects of adopting the Mediterranean diet, including reduced lipid peroxidation, high efficiency of oxidative repair, increased antioxidant defense system, and reduced mitochondrial generation rate.

Maintains Blood Sugar Level

The Mediterranean diet focuses on healthy carbs and whole grains. It has a lot of significant benefits. Consumption of whole-grain foods, like buckwheat, quinoa, and wheat berries instead of refined foods, helps you maintain blood sugar levels that ultimately gives you enough energy for the whole day.

Enhances Cognitive Health

The Mediterranean diet helps in preserving memory. It is one of the most useful steps for Alzheimer's treatment and dementia. Cognitive disorders occur when our brains do not get sufficient dopamine, which is a crucial chemical vital for mood regulation, thought processing, and body movements. Healthy fats like olive oil and nuts are good at fighting cognitive decline, mostly an age-related issue. They help counter some harmful impacts of the free radicals, inflammation, and toxins caused by having a low diet. The Mediterranean diet proves to be beneficial in decreasing

the risk of Alzheimer's to a great extent. Foods like yogurt help in having a healthy gut that improves mood, cognitive functioning, and memory.

Better Endurance Level

Mediterranean diet helps in fat loss and maintains muscle mass. It improves physical performance and enhances endurance levels. Research done on mice has shown positive results in these aspects. It also improves the health of our tissues in the long-term. The growth hormone also offers increased levels as a result of the Mediterranean diet. Which ultimately helps in improving metabolism and body composition.

Keeps You Agile

The nutrients from the Mediterranean diet reduces your risk of muscle weakness and frailty. It increases longevity. When your risk of heart disease reduces, it also reduces the risk of early death. It also strengthens your bones. Certain compounds found in olive oil help in preserving bone density. It helps increase the maturation and proliferation of the bone cells—dietary patterns of the Mediterranean diet help prevent osteoporosis.

Healthy Sleep Patterns

Our eating habits have a considerable impact on sleepiness and wakefulness. Some Mediterranean diet believers have reported an improved sleeping pattern as a result of changing their eating patterns. It has a considerable impact on your sleep because they regulate the circadian rhythm that determines our sleep patterns. If you have a regulated and balanced circadian rhythm, you will fall asleep quite quickly. You will also feel refreshed when you wake up. Another theory states that having the last meal will help you digest the food way before sleep. Digestion works best when you are upright.

Apart from focusing on plant-based eating, the Mediterranean diet philosophy emphasizes variety and moderation, living a life with perfect harmony with nature, valuing relationships in life, including sharing and enjoying meals, and having an entirely active lifestyle. The Mediterranean diet is at the crossroads. With the traditions and culture of three millennia, the Mediterranean diet lifestyle made its way to the medical world a long time ago. It has progressively recognized and became one of the successful and healthiest patterns that lead to a healthy lifestyle.

Besides metabolic, cardiovascular, cognitive, and many other benefits, this diet improves your life quality. Therefore, it is recommended today by many medical professionals worldwide. Efforts are being made in both non--Mediterranean and Mediterranean populations to make everyone benefit from the fantastic network of eating habits and patterns that began in old-time and which became a medical recommendation for a healthy lifestyle.

What to Eat and what to avoid

Fruits and vegetables: Mediterranean diet is one of the plant-based diet plans. Fresh fruits and vegetables contain a large number of vitamins, nutrients, fibers, minerals, and antioxidants

Fruits: Apple, berries, grapes, peaches, fig, grapefruit, dates, melon, oranges and pears.

Vegetables: Spinach, Brussels sprout, kale, tomatoes, kale, summer squash, onion, cauliflower, peppers, cucumbers, turnips, potatoes, sweet potatoes, and parsnips.

Seeds and nuts: Seeds and nuts are rich in monounsaturated fats and omega- 3 fatty acids.

Seeds: pumpkin seeds, flax seeds, sesame seeds, and sunflower seeds. Nuts: Almond, hazelnuts, pistachios, cashews, and walnuts.

Whole grains: Whole grains are high in fibers and they are not processed so they do not contain unhealthy fats like trans-fats compare to processed ones.

Whole grains: Wheat, quinoa, rice, barley, oats, rye, and brown rice. You can also use bread and pasta which is made from whole grains.

Fish and seafood: Fish are the rich source of omega-3 fatty acids and proteins. Eating fish at least once a week is recommended here. The healthiest way to consume fish is to grill it. Grilling fish taste good and never need extra oil.

Fish and seafood: salmon, trout, clams, mackerel, sardines, tuna and shrimp.

Legumes: Legumes (beans) are a rich source of protein, vitamins, and fibers. Regular consumption of beans helps to reduce the risk of diabetes, cancer and heart disease.

Legumes: Kidney beans, peas, chickpeas, black beans, fava beans, lentils, and pinto beans.

Spices and herbs: Spices and herbs are used to add the taste to your meal.

Spices and herbs: mint, thyme, garlic, basil, cinnamon, nutmeg, rosemary, oregano and more.

Healthy fats: Olive oil is the main fat used in the Mediterranean diet. It helps to reduce the risk of inflammatory disorder, diabetes, cancer, and heart- related disease. It also helps to increase HDL (good cholesterol) levels and decrease LDL (bad cholesterol) levels into your body. It also helps to lose weight.

Fats: Olive oil, avocado oil, walnut oil, extra virgin olive oil, avocado, and olives.

Dairy: Moderate amounts of dairy products are allowed during the Mediterranean diet. The dairy product contains high amounts of fats.

Dairy: Greek yogurt, skim milk and cheese.

Food to avoid

Refined grains: Refined grains are not allowed in a Mediterranean diet. It raises your blood sugar level. Refined grains like white bread, white rice, and pasta.

Refined oils: Oils like vegetable oils, cottonseed oils, and soybean oils are completely avoided from the Mediterranean diet. It raises your LDL (bad cholesterol) level.

Added Sugar: Added sugar is not allowed in the Mediterranean diet. These types of artificial sugars are found in table sugar, soda, chocolate, ice cream, and candies. It raises your blood sugar level.

You should consume only natural sugars in the Mediterranean diet.

Processed foods: Generally Processed foods come in boxes. Its low-fat food should not be eaten during the diet. It contains a high amount of trans-fats. Mediterranean diet is all about to eat fresh and natural food.

Trans-fat and saturated fats: In this category of food contains butter and margarine.

Processed Meat: Mediterranean diet does not allow to use of processed meat such as bacon, hot dogs and sausage.

Soups & Salads

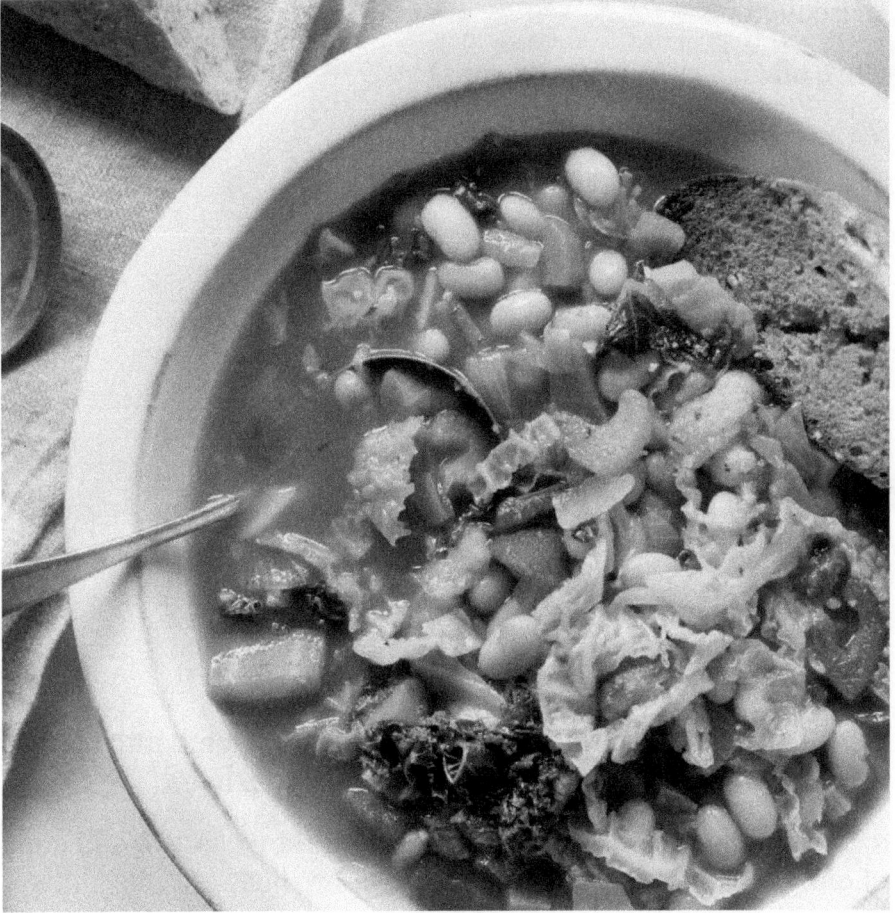

Greek Easter Lamb Soup With Egg Lemon Sauce

Servings: 3

Ingredients

Olive oil (1/2 cup) Water (5 cups)

Two pounds, bone in lamb

Ten green onions, chopped

Two bunches dill, chopped

One head romaine lettuce, chopped very thin

Juice of three lemons

Three eggs

Directions:

1.   Chop dill, onions and lettuce.

2.   Trim fat from the lamb and discard. Cut lamb into pieces about one inch large but do not throw away the bone.

3.   Set a large-sized stock skillet on the stove. Add a half cup of oil. Warm it over a medium temperature heat.

4.   Drop in lamb and bone, cooking them for ten minutes, stirring consistently.

5.   Toss in the green onions and cook for another three minutes.

6.   Add five cups of water and boil before allowing to simmer covered for thirty minutes.

7.   Add lettuce, dill, salt, and pepper. Simmer for one hour.

8.   Mix the eggs and lemon juice in a mixing bowl.

9.   While whisking, add two ladlesful of broth from the soup very slowly into the egg mixture. Make sure to keep whisking the whole time.

10.   Remove skillet from the stove.

11.   Pour in sauce and immediately stir the soup.

Tuscan White Bean Soup With Sausage And Kale

Servings: 6

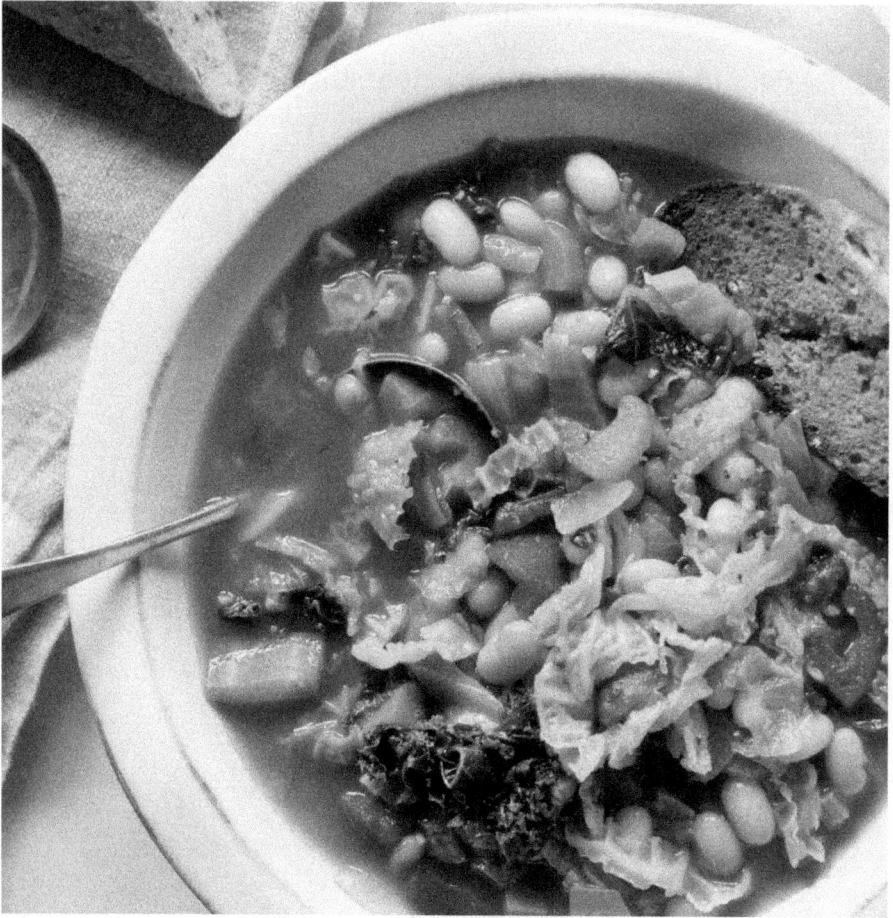

Ingredients

hot or sweet Italian sausage (One pound) One onion

One carrot

Dried rosemary (1 teaspoon) One stalk celery

Two cloves garlic

One half pound of kale stems removed and chopped Chicken broth (4 cups)

One can cannelloni beans rinsed and drained 28 ounce Pepper (¼ teaspoon)

Salt

Extra virgin olive oil (¼ cup) One bay leaf

Shredded parmesan (½ cup)

Directions:

1.   Cut sausage into small pieces. Chop onion, carrot, celery, garlic, and kale.

2.   Over a medium temperature heat in a soup skillet, cook the sausage until browned.

3.   Toss in onion, celery, garlic, carrot, and garlic to skillet, cooking for another three minutes.

4.   Add kale to the skillet, stirring gently, cooking until it begins to wilt.

5.   Add broth, beans, rosemary, and bay leaf.

6.   Boil, covering the skillet, then simmering for thirty minutes, stirring occasionally.

Zucchini Basil Soup With Lemon

Servings: 4

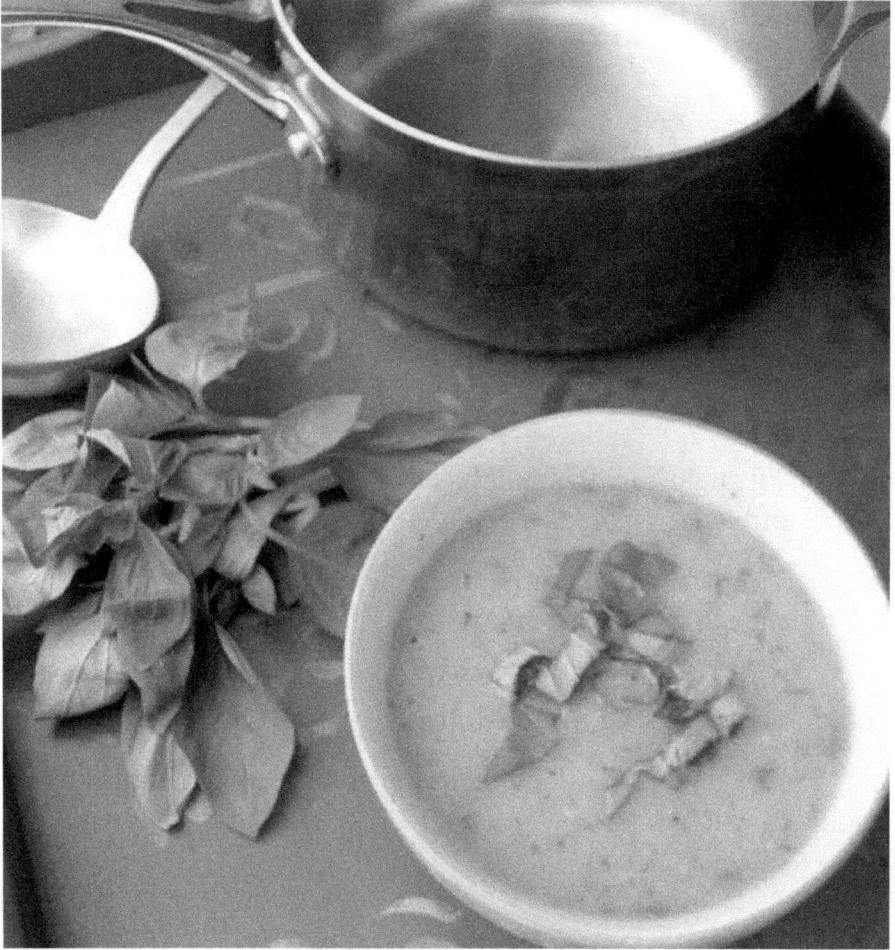

Ingredients

Olive oil (2 tablespoons) One medium onion

Three to four cloves garlic Four medium zucchini Chicken broth (3 cups) Zest of one lemon

Loosely packed basil (1/2 cup) Basil leaves, chopped

Sea salt and pepper

Lemon wedges Parmesan cheese, grated Greek yogurt

Directions:

1.   Chop onion and garlic. Peel and chop zucchini.

2.   In a medium-sized stock skillet, add oil and onion and cook for about five minutes.

3.   Toss in garlic, cooking mixture for another minute or so, stirring frequently. Throw in the zucchini, cooking for five minutes, stirring frequently.

4.   Add in zest and broth and boil. Before reducing temperature and simmer until zucchini is nice and tender and cooked all the way through. Then stir in basil.

5.   Pour into blender, blend well and return to stock skillet.

6.   Sprinkle with the pepper and salt.

Orange Lentil Soup

Servings: 4

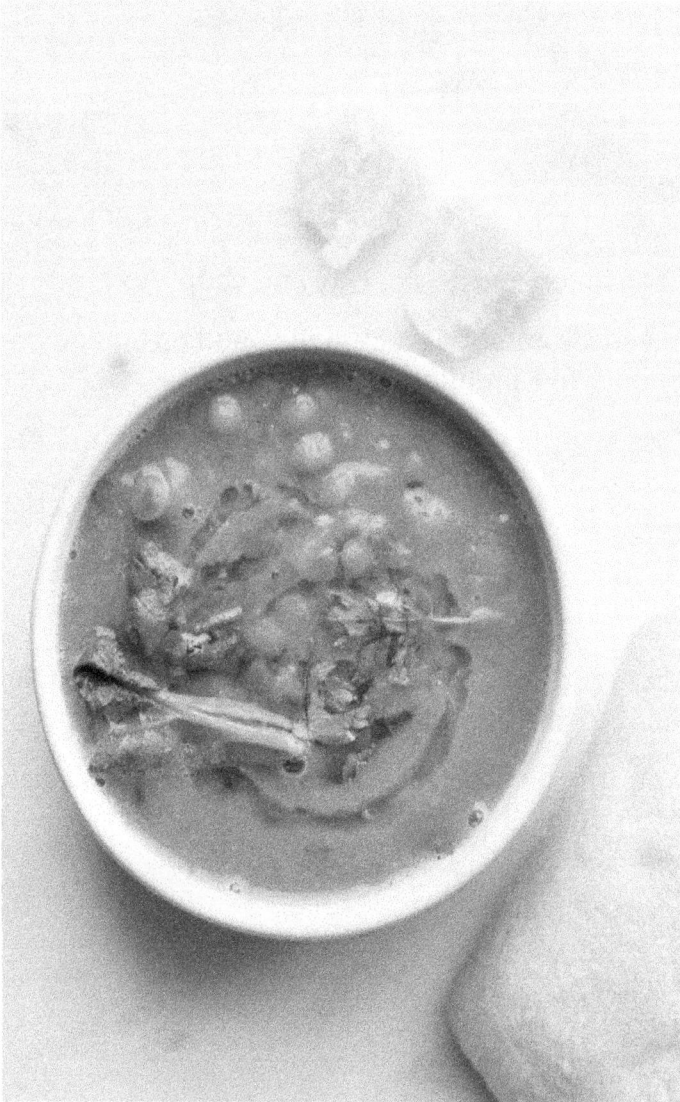

Ingredients

Extra virgin olive oil (1 cup)

One pound washed lentils

Two cloves garlic

Tomato paste (2 tablespoons)

One onion

Water (6 cups)

Three carrots

Two orange slices

One bay leaf

Directions:

1.   Mince garlic cloves. Grate onion and carrots. Peel orange slices.

2.   Boil lentils and six cups water in a skillet for fifteen minutes.

3.   Drop in the remainder of the ingredients and reduce temperature to a low boil for a half hour or until the lentils are soft.

Shrimp & Cod Stew In Tomato-Saffron Broth

Servings: 4

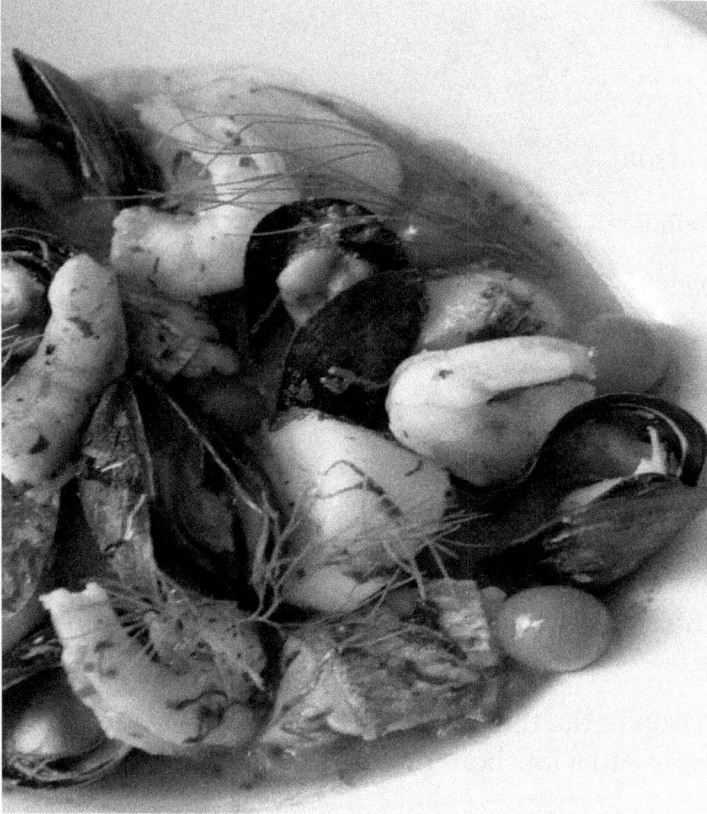

Ingredients:

Pepper (1/4 teaspoon)

Olive oil (2 tablespoons)

One large onion

Three garlic cloves

Dried thyme (1 tablespoon)

Ground turmeric (1 teaspoon)

Whole kernel corn (1 cup)

Two bay leaves

Two cans diced tomatoes (14-1/2 ounces each)

Cod fillet (One pound)

Large shrimp (One pound, uncooked)

Water (2 cups)

One can (14-1/2 ounces) vegetable broth

One baby spinach package (about 6 ounces)

Lemon wedges

Directions:

1.   Heat up your olive oil on medium temperature heat in a regular skillet.

2.   Mince the thyme and cloves and chop the onion. Chop the fish in one-inch cube shapes. Peel and devein shrimp.

3.   Add onions, stirring until soft and cooked.

4.   Mix in garlic, thyme, saffron and bay leaves and cook the mixture for a minute. Pour in tomatoes, fish, broth, water, shrimp, corn and pepper.

5.   Boil the mixture, then quickly reduce the heat simmering

6.   Add in the spinach during the final stages of cooking. Remove

Tuscan White Bean Stew

Servings: 4

Ingredients

Directions:

and discard the bay leaves and serve with lemon wedges.

Olive oil (1 tablespoon) Two cloves garlic

One slice of whole-grain bread For soup:

Dried cannellini or other white beans, (2 cups) Black pepper (1/4 teaspoon)

One bay leaf

Salt (1/2 teaspoon) Yellow onion (1 cup) Three carrots

Olive oil (2 tablespoons) Six cloves garlic

Water (6 cups)

Chopped fresh rosemary (1 tablespoon) Vegetable stock or broth (1 1/2 cups)

1.   Quarter garlic. Cut whole grain bread into half-inch cubes.

2.   Rinse and drain beans.

3.   Chop onion, carrots and six cloves of garlic. Quarter two cloves of garlic for croutons.

4.   Using a pan, heat up oil on a medium. Drop in the quartered

garlic, cooking for about one minute.

5.   Pull pan from the heat, letting it stand for ten minutes. Remove all cooked garlic pieces and throw them away.

6.   Bring skillet to medium heat.

7.   Stirring frequently, drop in bread cubes and cook for three to five minutes. Pour into a small bowl, setting aside for now.

8.   Combine the water, beans, a quarter teaspoon of the salt and the bay leaf. Use a medium sized skillet. Boil then pull down the heat to low temperature and cover the skillet. Allow to simmer until beans are nice and tender, which should take about 60 to 75 minutes.

9.   Drain all the beans, saving about a half a cup of liquid from the beans. Throw away the bay leaf.

10.   Put beans into a bowl.

11.   Combine saved bean liquid and a half cup of the cooked beans in a small sized bowl. Mash into a textured cream. Stir the cooked beans together with the bean paste.

12.   Return the cooking skillet to the stovetop, adding olive oil and cook over medium heat.

13.   Add in onions and carrots, cooking for five to

six minutes.

14.   Drop in the garlic. Stir in the rest of the salt,

stock, the rosemary, pepper, bean mixture, and boil. Bring heat back down and allow to simmer until heated through.

15. Pour into serving bowls, add croutons and garnish if desired.

Cauliflower Soup With Cream

Servings: 6

Ingredients:

Chopped garlic cloves - 2 Chicken stock – 2 cups

Large head cauliflower – 1 (cut into florets) Pepper and salt to taste

Rosemary sprig – 1 Chopped shallot - 1 Heavy cream – ½ cup Olive oil – 2 tbsps.

Feta cheese for serving – 3 oz.

Directions:

1.   Stir in a soup skillet garlic, shallow and heated oil. Add pepper, cauliflower, rosemary sprig, salt and stock after cooking for 2 minutes.

2.   On low heat, remove the rosemary after cooking for 15 minutes and stir in the cream.

3.   Use immersion blender to puree the soup and serve the soup chilled or warm, top it with crumbled feta cheese.

Gorgeous Kale Soup made with white bean

Servings: 8

Ingredients:

Drained white beans – 1 can Shredded kale – 1 bunch Chopped shallot – 1

Water – 6 cups

Chopped garlic cloves - 2 Diced carrots - 2

Lemon juice – 2 tbsps Diced tomatoes – 1 can Chopped red pepper - 1 Vegetable stock – 2 cups Pepper and salt to taste

Directions:

Olive oil – 2 tbsps Diced celery stalk - 1

1.   Stir in a soup skillet celery, garlic, carrots, shallot, red pepper and heated oil. Soften it by cooking for 2 minutes.

2.   Add other Ingredients: and season with pepper and salt.

3.   On low heat, cook the soup for 30 minutes.

4.   Enjoy the soup as you serve it chill or warm.

Refreshing Chorizo Soup

Servings: 6

Ingredients:

Vegetable stock – 2 cups Olive oil – 2 tbsps Chopped shallot - 1

Cored and diced red bell peppers - 1 Diced carrots - 2

Cored and diced yellow bell pepper - 1 Drained white beans – 1 can

Chopped garlic clove - 1 Diced tomatoes – 1 can Water – 6 cups

Thyme sprig - 1 Chopped red pepper - 1 Pepper and salt to taste Sliced chorizo links - 2

Directions:

1.   In a soup skillet, pour the oil and heat it

2.   Cook for 5 minutes after stirring in the chorizo links.

3.   Then add all other Ingredients: and season with pepper and salt.

4.   On low heat, cook the soup for 25 minutes.   Serve the soup

warm when it's done.

Mediterranean Bean and Sausage soup

Servings: 4

Ingredients:

Directions:

Olive oil 2 tablespoons

A can of drained black beans Juiced tomato; 1 cup

4 cups of water

1 pound of sliced chicken sausage 2 cups of chicken stalk

1 chopped celery stalk 2 sliced cloves

1   can of drained kidney beans 1 sliced carrot

2   peeled and sliced tomatoes A rosemary sprig

1 bay leaf

A sweet onion; diced Pepper and salt to taste

1.   Get a soup skillet and heat your olive oil, then pour in your sausage and cook for 5 minutes.

2.   Now, add all other ingredients.

3.   Add pepper and salt to taste and cook for 25 minutes.

4.   Serve and enjoy when cooled

Mediterranean Chicken Soup

Servings: 5

Ingredients:

2 sliced cloves

2 peeled and sliced tomatoes

A bay leaf

1 juiced lemon

1 sweet onion; diced 1 cubed zucchini

Water; 4 cups

½ teaspoon of capers; sliced

½ teaspoon of oregano; dried Dried basil; 1 teaspoon

½ cup of orzo Chicken stock; 2 cups

1 pound of chicken drumsticks

1 chopped and cored green bell pepper 1 chopped and cored red bell pepper Pepper and salt to taste

Directions:

1.   Get a soup skillet and add your vegetable, stock, herbs, chicken, bay leaf and water together, then add pepper and salt to taste and cook on low heat for 25 minutes.

2.   Now add your lemon juice and cook again for 5 minutes.

3.   Serve and enjoy your warm soup.

Chicken Sausage Minestrone

Servings: 4

Ingredients:

4 sliced chicken sausage

4 tomatoes sliced and peeled 2 chopped cloves

½ pound of diced green beans 2 sliced carrots

A dubbed zucchini Olive oil 2 tablespoons 1 diced sweet onion

½ cup of green peas 1 sliced celery stalk

2 cups of vegetable stalk

½ cup of marjoram Water 6 cups

½ teaspoon of oregano

½ teaspoon of basil Pepper and salt to taste

Directions:

1.   Get a soup skillet and heat the oil, then pour in your chicken sausage and some diced onion, then cook for 5 minutes.

2.   Now, add in your tomatoes, carrot, cloves, onion and celery and wait till it's cooked for another 10 minutes then add your remaining ingredients.

3.   Add pepper and salt to taste, then cook for 20 minutes.

4.   Serve and enjoy your soup when warm.

Delicious Meatball Soup for the Spanish

Servings: 8

Ingredients:

Water – 6 cups

Crushed tomatoes – 1 can

Egg - 1

Olive oil – 2 tbsps

Diced celery stalk - 1

Chopped onion - 1

Cored and diced red bell peppers – 2

Vegetable stock – 2 cups

Diced carrots - 2

Pound ground veal - 1

Chopped parsley – 2 tbsps

Chopped garlic cloves - 2

Pepper and salt to taste

Directions:

1.   In a soup skillet, heat the oil and stir in the garlic, stock, bell peppers, onions, carrots, water and celery.

2.   Bring to a boiling after seasoning with pepper and salt. In a bowl, mix egg, veal and parsley in the meantime.

3.   Then boil them in boiling liquid after forming small meatballs.

4.   Adjust the taste with pepper and salt after adding the tomatoes.

5.   For 20 minutes, cook on heat that is very low.

6.   Best served fresh and warm.

Special Orzo Soup

Servings: 8

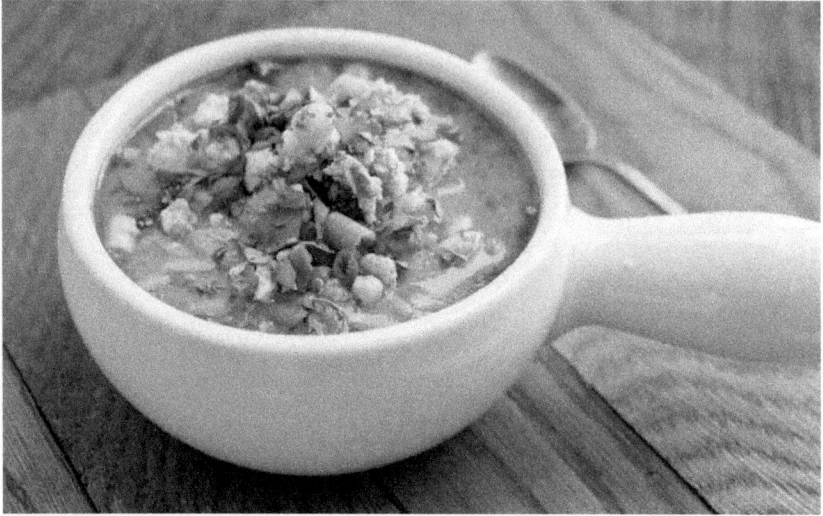

Ingredients:

Orzo – ¼ cup

Vegetable stock – 2 cups Lemon juice – 2 tbsps

Cored and diced yellow bell pepper - 1 Extra virgin olive oil – 2 tbsps Chopped shallots - 2

Baby spinach – 4 cups Green peas – 1 cup

Cored and diced green bell pepper - 1 Water – 4 cups

Chopped garlic cloves - 2 Pepper and salt to taste

Directions:

1.   In a soup skillet, heat the oil and stir in the garlic and shallots.

2.   Add other Ingredients: after cooking it for 2 minutes and season with pepper and salt.

3.   On low heat, cook it for 25 minutes.

4.   Best served chilled or warm.

Cozy Cod Soup

Servings: 8

Ingredients:

Olive oil - 2 tbsp.

Carrot - 1, sliced

Red bell pepper - 1, cored and diced

Shallots - 2, chopped

Celery – 1 stalk, sliced

Garlic cloves - 2, chopped

Marjoram - ½ tsp.

Marjoram - ½ tsp.

Potatoes - 1 ½ lbs., peeled and cubed

Tomatoes - 1 cup, diced

Cod fillets - 4, cubed

Bay leaf - 1 leaf

Thyme - 1 sprig

Water - 6 cups

Lemon juice - 2 tbsp.

Chicken stock - 2 cups

Salt and pepper - to taste

Directions:

1.   Heat olive oil in a skillet and add garlic, shallots, bell pepper, celery, and carrot.

2.   After cooking for 5 minutes you will add in bay leaf, marjoram, stock, tomatoes, water, potatoes, thyme, and marjoram.

3.   Add in salt and pepper to suit your taste and lower heat, cooking an additional 20 minutes.

4.   Place cod in the skillet, add lemon juice and cook for 5 more minutes. Serve right away.

One Hour Fennel Soup

Servings: 6

 Ingredients:

Leek - 1, sliced

Garlic cloves - 3,

chopped Olive oil - 2 tbsp.

Shallot - 1,

chopped Stalk of celery – 1,

diced Carrot - 1, diced

Fennel bulb - 1, sliced

Vegetable stock - 2 cups

Potato - 1, peeled and cubed

Tomatoes - 2, peeled and diced

Harissa powder - ¼ tsp.

Lemon juice - 1 tbsp.

Cumin powder - ¼ tsp.

Water - 1 cup

Salt and pepper - to taste

Thyme - 1 sprig

Directions:

1.   Add olive oil to skillet and heat. After oil is heated, add carrot, celery, leek, fennel, shallot and garlic and cook for 5 minutes.

2.   Add in the rest of the Ingredients: above (salt and pepper to suit your taste) and cook for an additional few minutes until vegetables are well cooked.

3.   This soup is delicious warm or chilled.

Arugula & Brown Rice Salad
Servings: 5

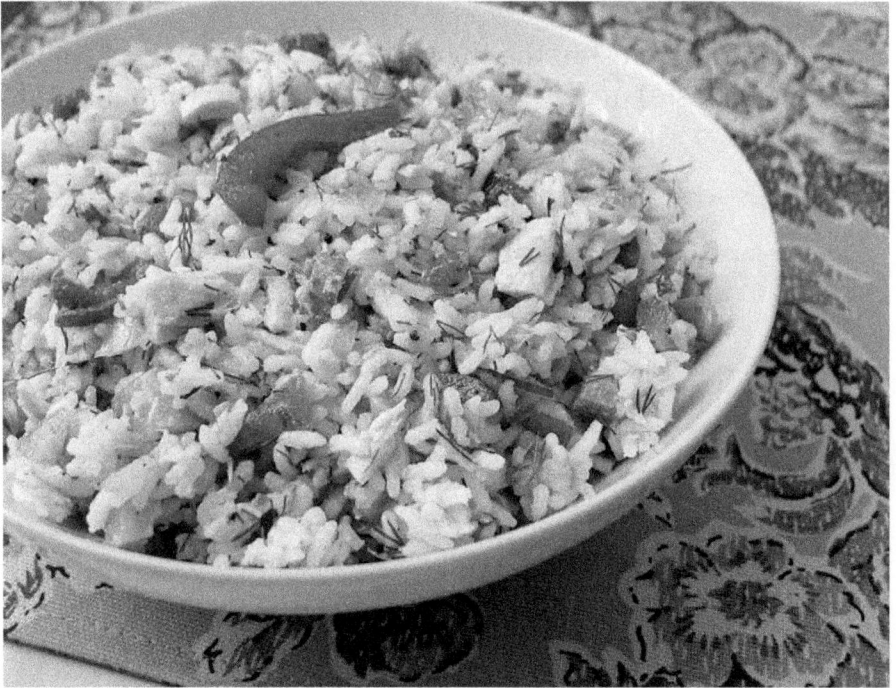

Ingredients

- Dried cherries or cranberries (1/2 cup)
- One package ready-to-serve brown rice
- One can garbanzo beans or chickpeas (15 ounces)
- Crumbled feta cheese (1 cup)
- Fresh arugula or baby spinach (7 cups)
- Basil leaves, torn (3/4 cup)

Dressing:

- Lemon juice (2 tablespoons)
- Pepper (1/8 teaspoon)
- Grated lemon peel (1/4 teaspoon)
- Salt (1/4 teaspoon)

- Olive oil (1/4 cup)

Directions:

1.   Rinse and drain chickpeas

2.   Heat rice according to package instructions. Transfer to a bowl and give it some time to cool down.

3.   Stir in the arugula, beans, cheese, basil, and cherries into the rice.

4.   Mix all of the ingredients together for the dressing. Drizzle carefully over the salad and toss evenly.

Roasted Bell Pepper Salad with Anchovy Dressing
Servings: 4

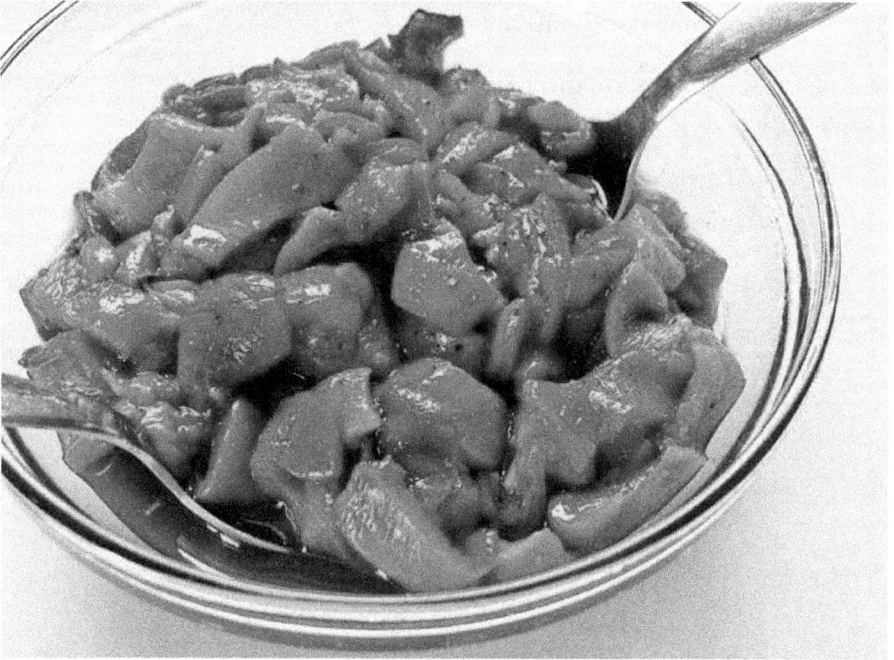

Ingredients:

- 8 roasted red bell peppers, sliced
- 2 tablespoons pine nuts
- 1 cup cherry tomatoes, halved
- 2 tablespoons chopped parsley
- 4 anchovy fillets
- 1 lemon, juiced
- 1 garlic clove
- 1 tablespoon extra-virgin olive oil
- Salt and pepper to taste

Directions:

1.   Combine the anchovy fillets, lemon juice, garlic and olive oil in a mortar and mix them well.

2.   Mix the rest of the ingredients in a salad bowl then drizzle in the dressing.

3.   Serve the salad as fresh as possible.

Pear Arugula Salad with Yogurt Dressing
Servings: 4

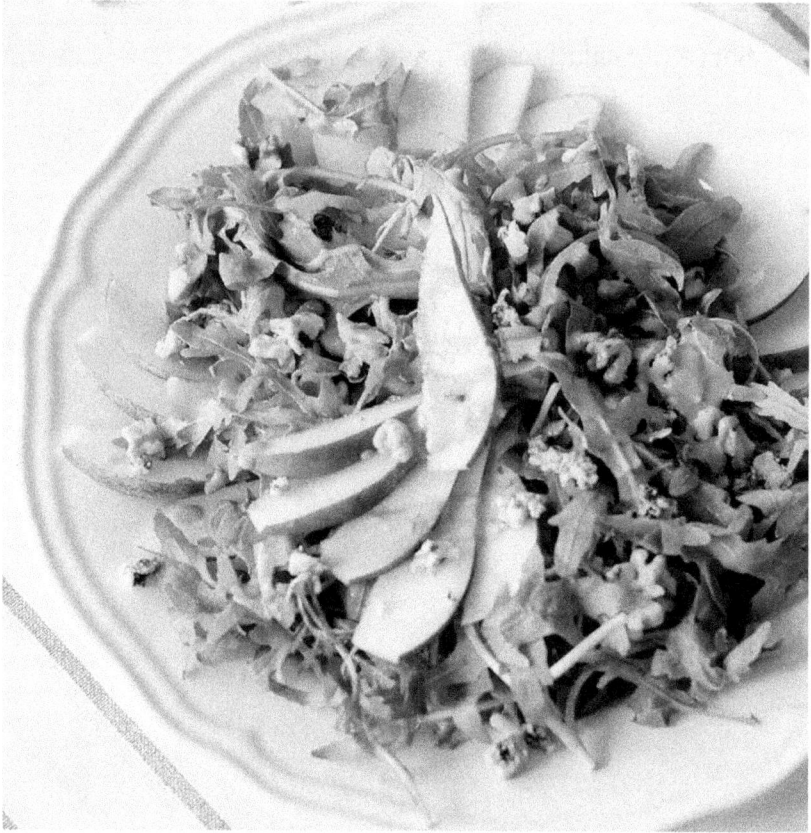

Ingredients:

- 4 cups arugula
- 4 pears, cored and sliced
- ½ cup walnuts, chopped
- 2 oz. blue cheese, crumbled
- ¼ cup plain yogurt

- tablespoon lemon juice
- tablespoons extra virgin olive oil Salt and pepper to taste

Directions:

1.   Combine the arugula, walnuts, pears and blue cheese in a salad bowl.

2.   For the dressing, mix the yogurt, lemon juice and oil in a jar. Add salt and pepper and shake well.

3.   Drizzle the dressing over the salad and serve right away.

Watermelon Feta Salad
Servings: 2

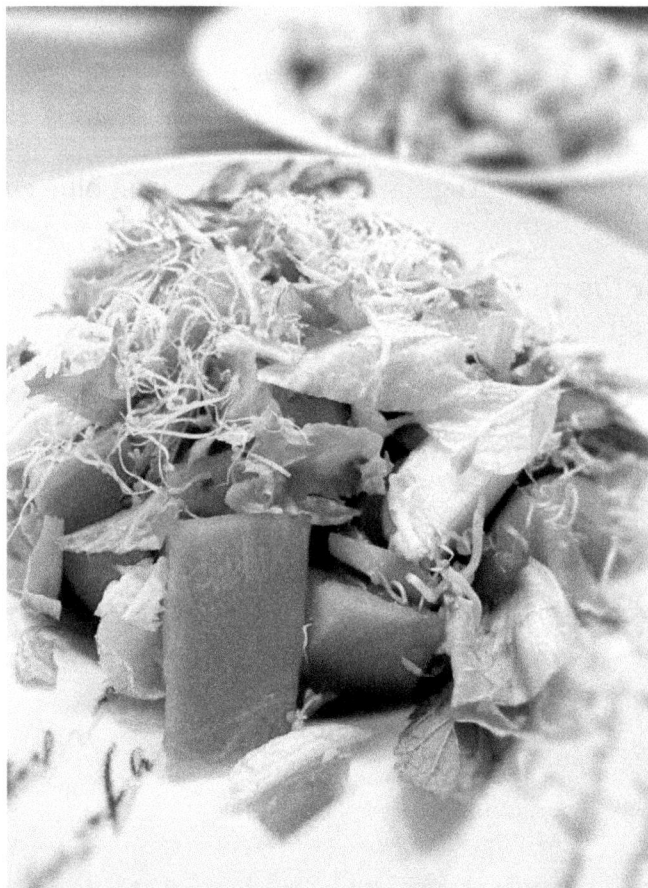

Ingredients:

- 16 oz. seedless watermelon, cubed
- 4 oz. feta cheese, crumbled
- 2 tablespoons extra virgin olive oil
- 1 teaspoon chopped thyme

Directions:

1. Combine the watermelon with the feta cheese in a bowl.
2. Drizzle with oil and sprinkle with thyme before serving.

Roasted Bell Pepper Eggplant Salad
Servings: 4

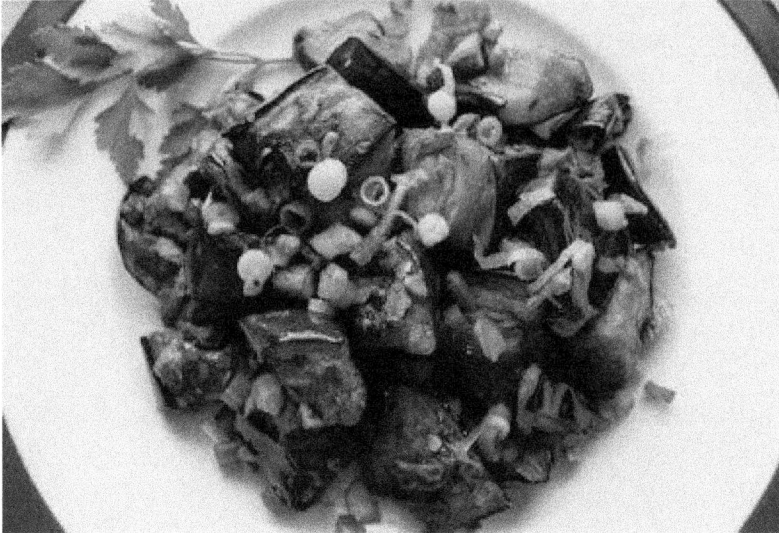

Ingredients:

- 1 eggplants, sliced
- 6 roasted red bell peppers, sliced
- 2 tablespoons tahini paste
- 1 pinch chili flakes
- Salt and pepper to taste

Directions:

1.   Combine all the ingredients in a bowl and season well with salt and pepper.

2.   Serve the salad fresh.

Pita Bread Bean Salad
Servings: 4

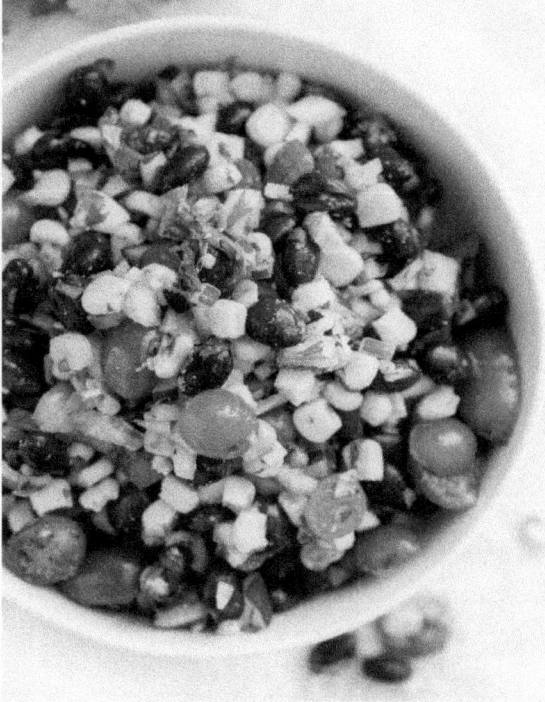

Ingredients:

- can red beans, drained
- 1 red onion, sliced
- tomatoes, cubed
- 2 pita breads, cubed
- tablespoons extra virgin olive oil
- 1 tablespoon balsamic vinegar
- Salt and pepper to taste

Directions:

1.   Combine the beans, red onion, pita bread, oil and vinegar in a salad bowl.

2.   Season with salt and pepper and serve the salad as fresh as possible.

Lettuce Cucumber Salad
Servings: 4

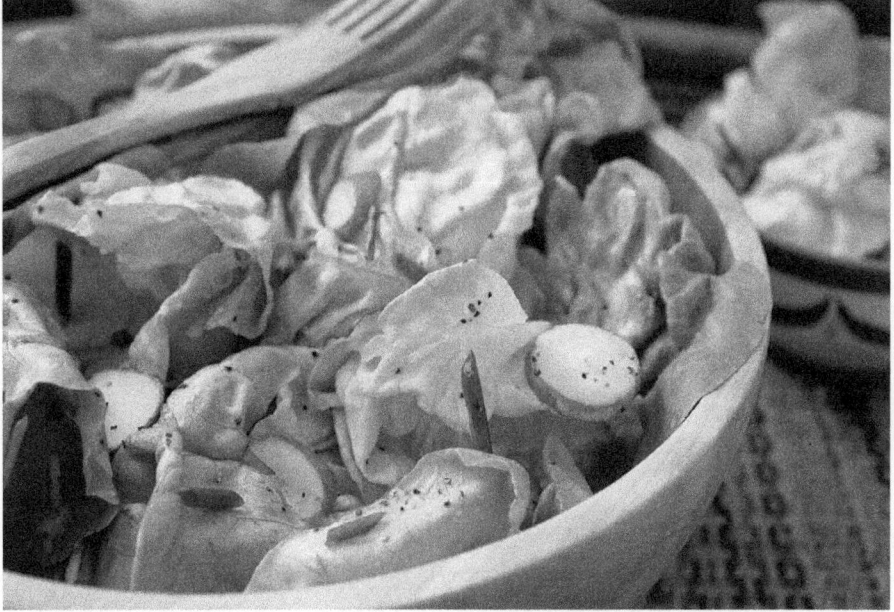

Ingredients:

- 1 lettuce head, shredded 4 cucumbers, sliced
- red pepper, chopped
- ¼ cup chopped parsley 1 teaspoon dried mint
- tablespoons extra virgin olive 1 lemon, juiced
- Salt and pepper to taste

Directions:

1. Combine the lettuce head, cucumber, red pepper, parsley and mint in a salad bowl.

2. Add the oil, lemon juice, salt and pepper and mix well.

3. Serve the salad fresh.

Provencal Summer Salad
Servings: 4

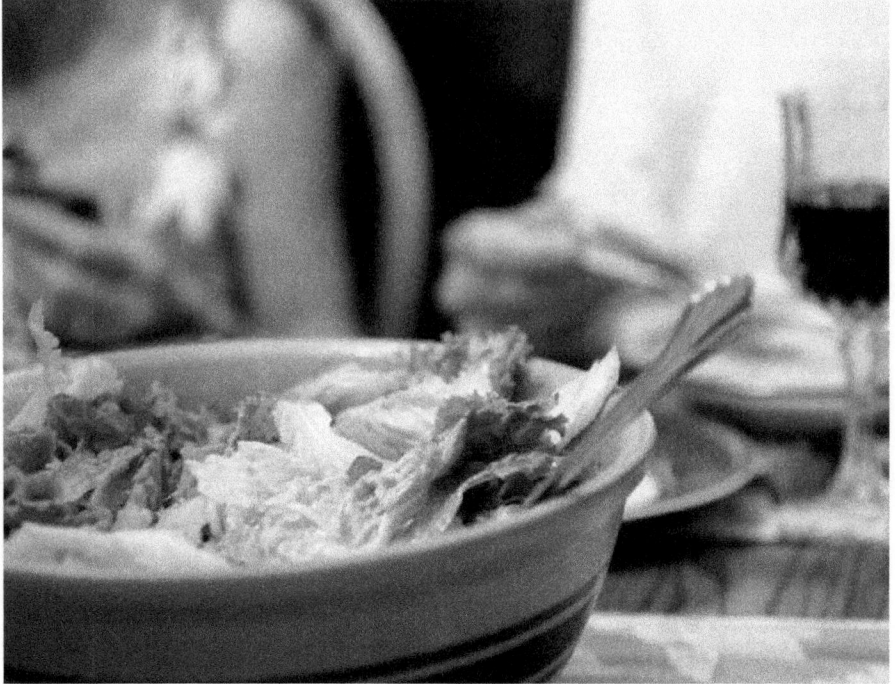

Ingredients:

- 1 zucchini, sliced
- eggplant, sliced
- red onions, sliced
- 2 tomatoes, sliced
- teaspoon dried mint
- 2 garlic cloves, minced
- 2   tablespoons balsamic vinegar
- Salt and pepper to taste

Directions:

1.   Season the zucchini, eggplant, onions and tomatoes with salt and pepper. Cook the vegetable slices on the grill until browned.

2.   Transfer the vegetables in a salad bowl then add the mint, garlic and vinegar.

3.   Serve the salad right away.

Red Beet Feta Salad
Servings: 4

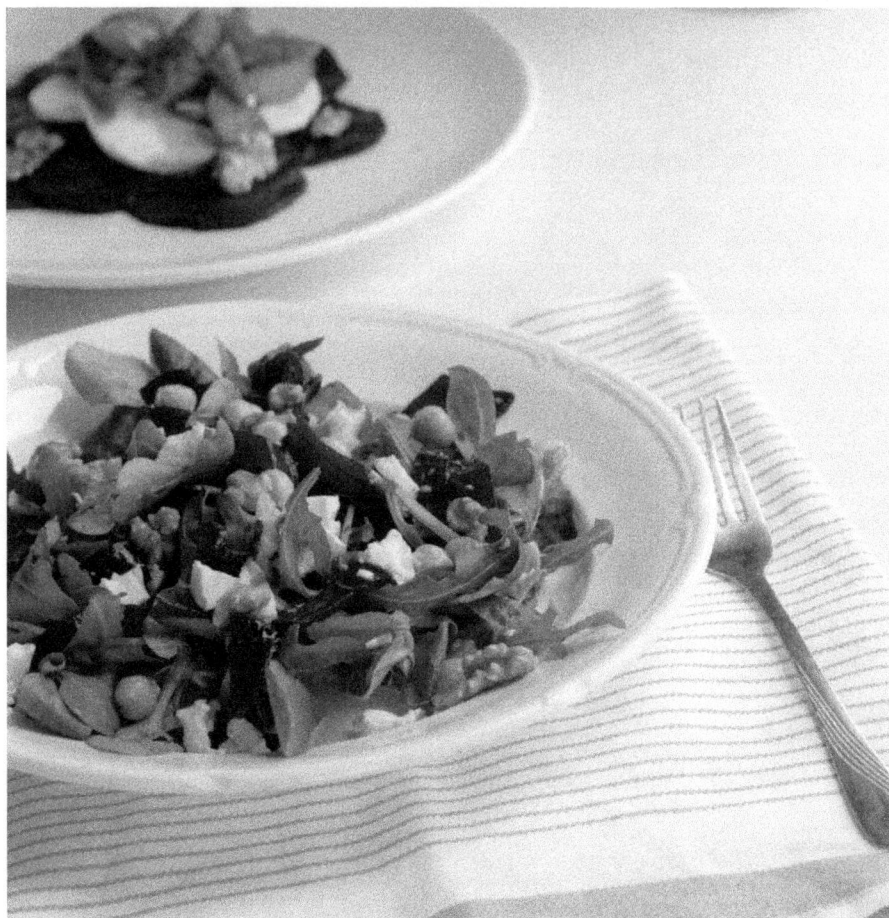

Ingredients:

- 6 red beets, cooked and peeled
- 3 oz. feta cheese, cubed
- 2 tablespoons extra virgin olive oil
- 2 tablespoons balsamic vinegar

Directions:

1. Combine the beets and feta cheese on a platter.

2. Drizzle with oil and vinegar and serve right away.

Spiced Parsley Salad
Servings: 2

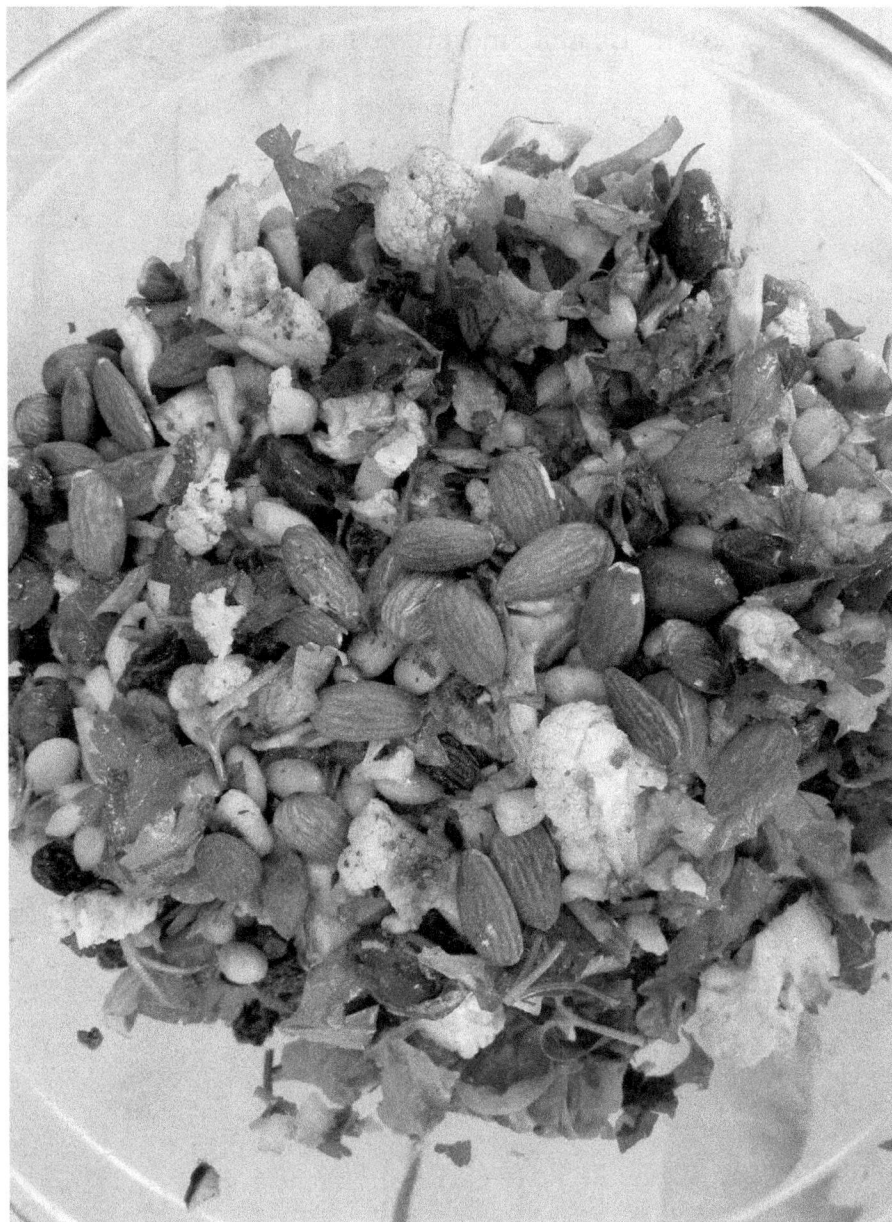

Ingredients:

- 2 cups chopped parsley
- ¼ cup chopped cilantro
- ¼ teaspoon cumin powder
- ¼ teaspoon chili powder
- ¼ teaspoon coriander seeds
- 1 tablespoon red wine vinegar Salt and pepper to taste

Directions:

1.   Combine the parsley, cilantro, spices and vinegar in a salad bowl.

2.   Add salt and pepper to taste and serve the salad as fresh as possible.

Tuscan Cabbage Salad
Servings: 4

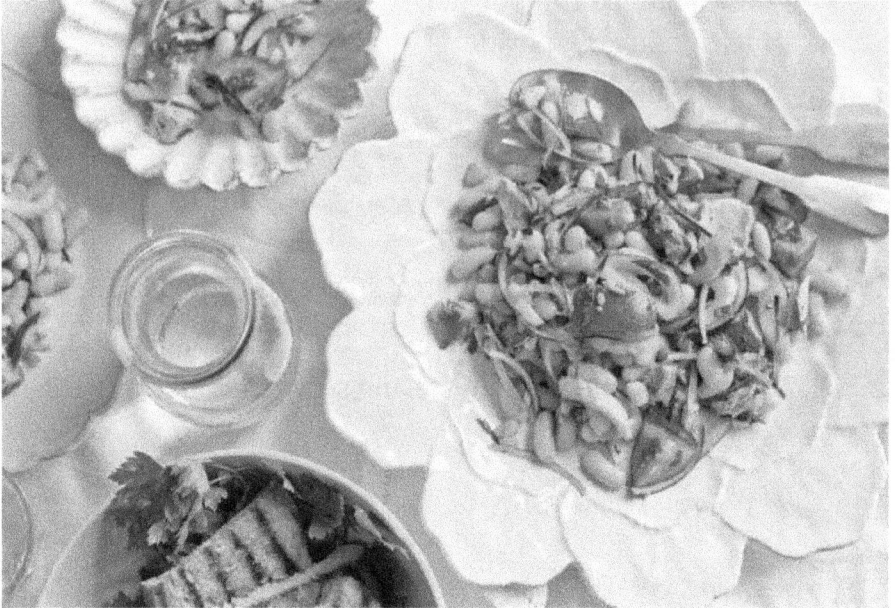

Ingredients:

1 head cabbage, shredded

½ cup chopped parsley 1 red pepper, chopped

1 green bell pepper, cored and sliced

1   yellow bell pepper, cored and sliced 1 red onion, sliced

Salt and pepper to taste

2   tablespoons apple cider vinegar 2 oz. pancetta, diced

Directions:

1.   Combine the cabbage, parsley, red pepper, bell peppers, red onion, salt and pepper in a salad bowl.

2.   Cook the pancetta in a frying pan until crisp then allow it to cool down and stir it into the salad.

3.   Serve the salad fresh.

Halibut Nicoise Salad
Servings: 4

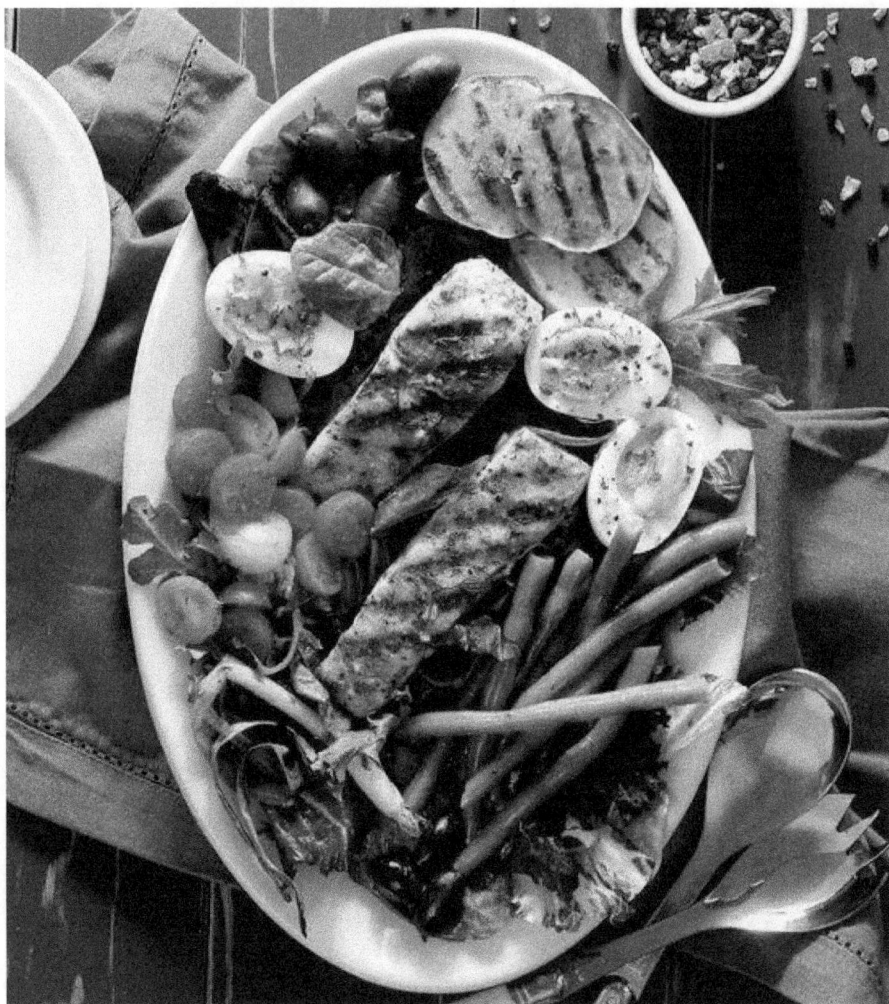

Ingredients:

- 2 halibut fillets
- teaspoon dried thyme Salt and pepper to taste 1 pound green beans
- hard-boiled eggs, cubed 2 anchovy fillets

- lemon, juiced
- garlic cloves
- teaspoon Dijon mustard
- tablespoons extra virgin olive oil

Directions:

1.   Season the halibut with thyme, salt and pepper and cook it on the grill until browned.

2.   When cooked, cut the halibut into small cubes.

3.   Pour a few cups of water in a large skillet and add a pinch of salt. Bring it to a boil then throw in the beans. Cook for 5 minutes then drain well and transfer in a salad bowl.

4.   Add the halibut and eggs.

5.   For the dressing, mix the anchovy fillets, mustard, lemon juice, garlic and oil in a mortar. Drizzle the dressing over the salad and mix well.

6.   Serve the salad as fresh as possible.

Stir-Fry Snap Pea Salad
Servings: 4

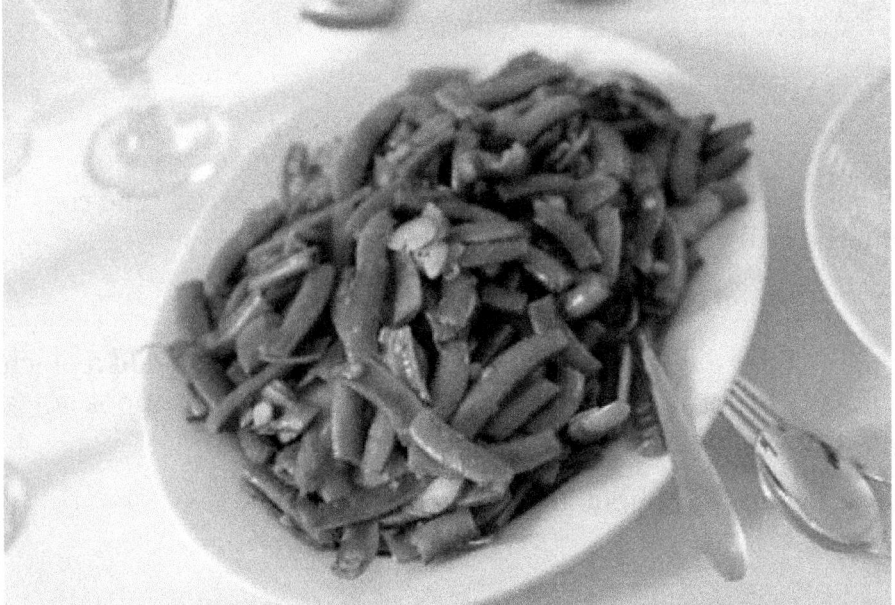

Ingredients:

- 3   tablespoons extra virgin olive oil
- 2 garlic cloves, minced
- 1 shallot, sliced
- pound snap peas
- tablespoons lemon juice
- 2 oz. grated Parmesan

Directions:

1.   Heat the oil in a frying pan then stir in the garlic and shallot. Cook for 1 minute until fragrant.

2.   Add the snap peas and cook briefly for 5-7 minutes.

3. When done, remove from heat and stir in the lemon juice.

4. Transfer into plates and top with Parmesan.

5. Serve the snap peas fresh.

Warm Shrimp and Arugula Salad
Servings: 4

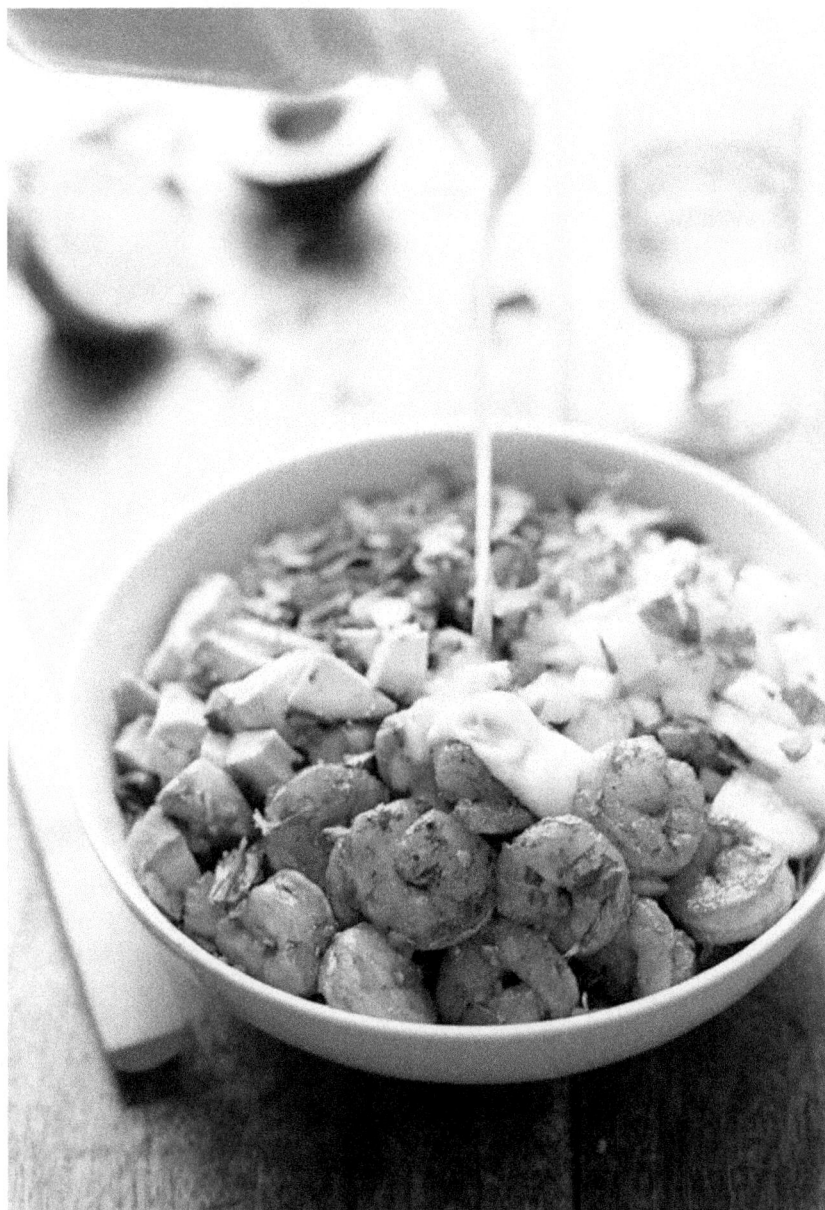

Ingredients:

- 2 tablespoons extra virgin olive oil 2 garlic cloves, minced
- 1 red pepper, sliced
- 1 pound fresh shrimps, peeled and deveined
- 1 orange, juiced
- Salt and pepper to taste 3 cups arugula

Directions:

1. Heat the oil in a frying pan and stir in the garlic and red pepper. Cook for 1 minute then add the shrimps.

2. Cook for 5 minutes then add the orange juice and cook for another 5 more minutes.

3. When done, spoon the shrimps and the sauce over the arugula.

4. Serve the salad fresh.

Bulgur Spinach Salad
Servings: 4

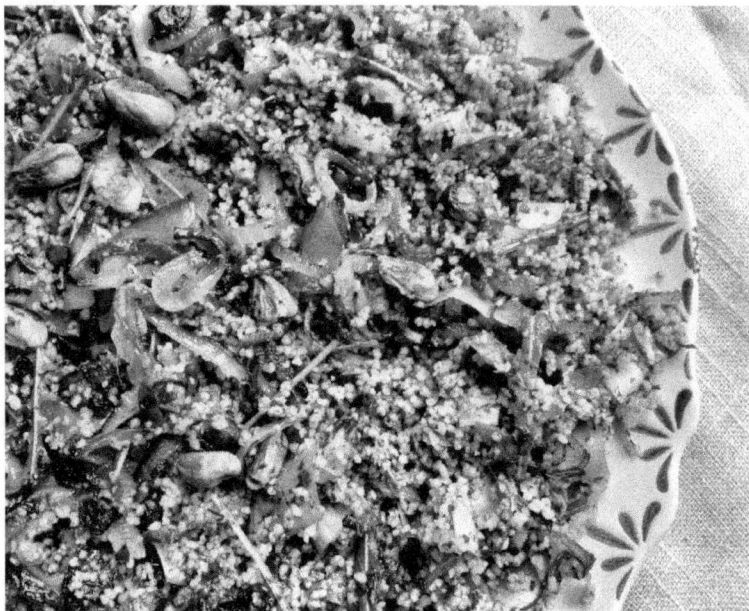

Ingredients:

- 2/3 cup bulgur
- 2 cups vegetable stock
- 8 oz. baby spinach
- 1 cup cherry tomatoes, halved
- 1 cucumber, diced
- ¼ cup dates, pitted and chopped
- 2 tablespoons sliced almonds
- 1 garlic clove, minced
- 1 tablespoon balsamic vinegar
- 1 tablespoon lemon juice
- Salt and pepper to taste
- 2   tablespoons mixed seeds

Directions:

1.   Combine the bulgur and stock in a saucepan and cook until all the liquid has been absorbed.

2.   Transfer the bulgur into a salad bowl and stir in the rest of the ingredients.

3.   Season with salt and pepper and mix well.

4.   Serve the salad as fresh as possible.

Artichoke Tuna Salad
Servings: 4

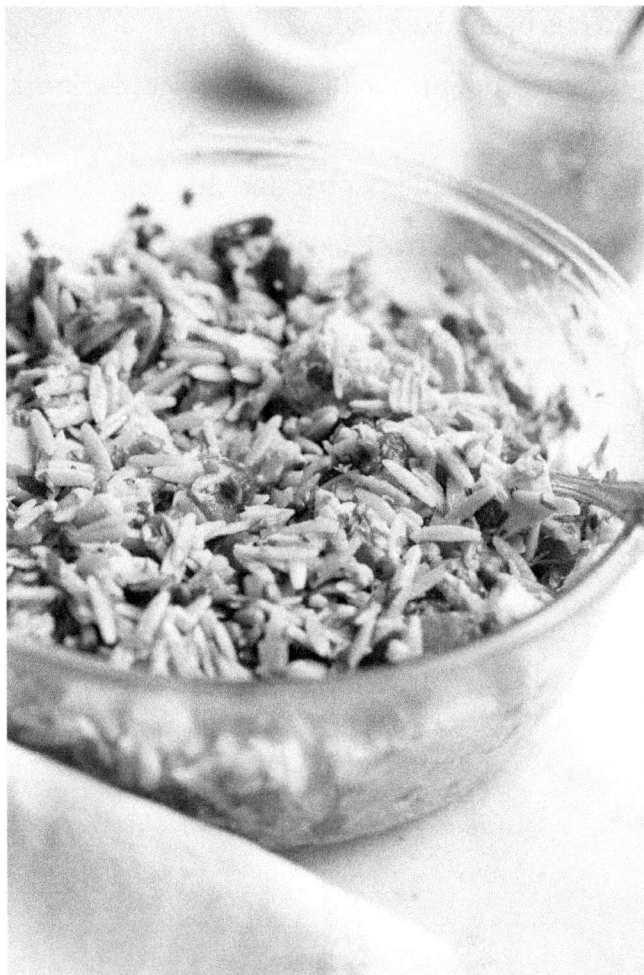

Ingredients:

- jar artichoke hearts, drained and chopped
- 1 can water tuna, drained
- arugula leaves

- tablespoons pine nuts
- ¼ cup green olives, sliced
- 1 lemon, juiced
- tablespoon Dijon mustard
- tablespoons extra virgin olive oil
- Salt and pepper to taste

Directions:

1.   Combine the artichoke hearts, tuna, green olives, arugula and pine nuts in a salad bowl.

2.   For the dressing, mix the lemon juice, mustard and oil.

3.   Drizzle the dressing over the salad and serve the salad as fresh as possible.

Grilled Sweet Potato Salad
Servings: 4

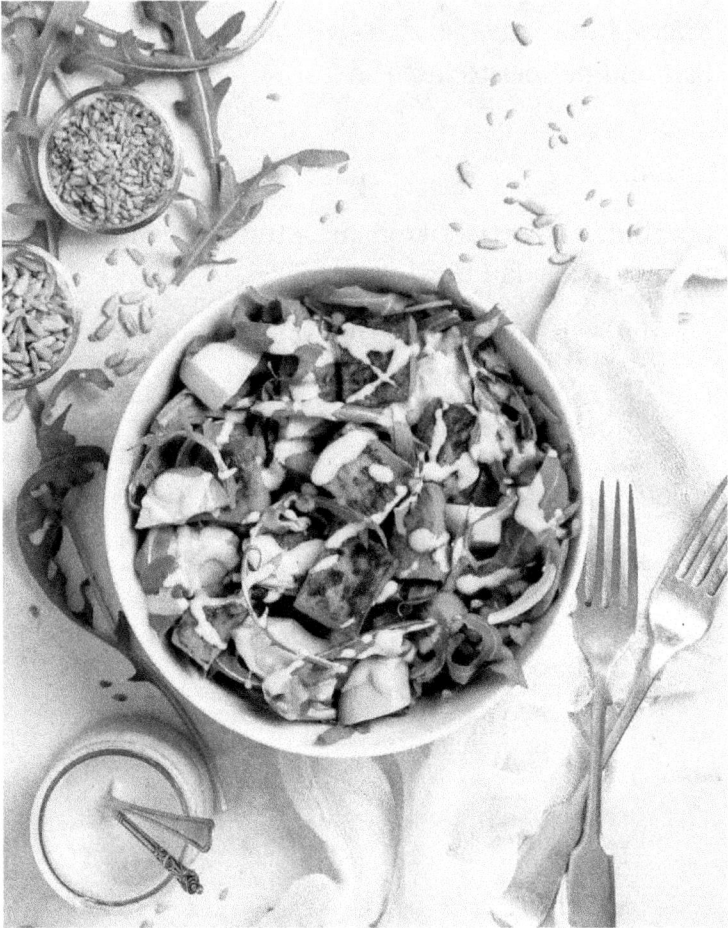

Ingredients:

- 2   sweet potatoes, finely sliced
- 3   tablespoons extra virgin olive oil
- 1 teaspoon sumac spices
- 2 tablespoons honey 1 teaspoon dried mint

- 3 cups mixed greens
- 1 tablespoon balsamic vinegar
- Salt and pepper to taste
- 1 pomegranate, seeded

Directions:

1.   Season the sweet potatoes with salt, pepper, sumac and mint then drizzle with oil and honey and mix well.

2.   Heat a grill pan over medium flame then place the sweet potatoes over the grill. Cook on each side until browned.

3.   Transfer the sweet potatoes in a salad bowl then stir in the mixed greens and pomegranate seeds.

4.   Serve the salad fresh.

Chickpea Salad
Servings: 4

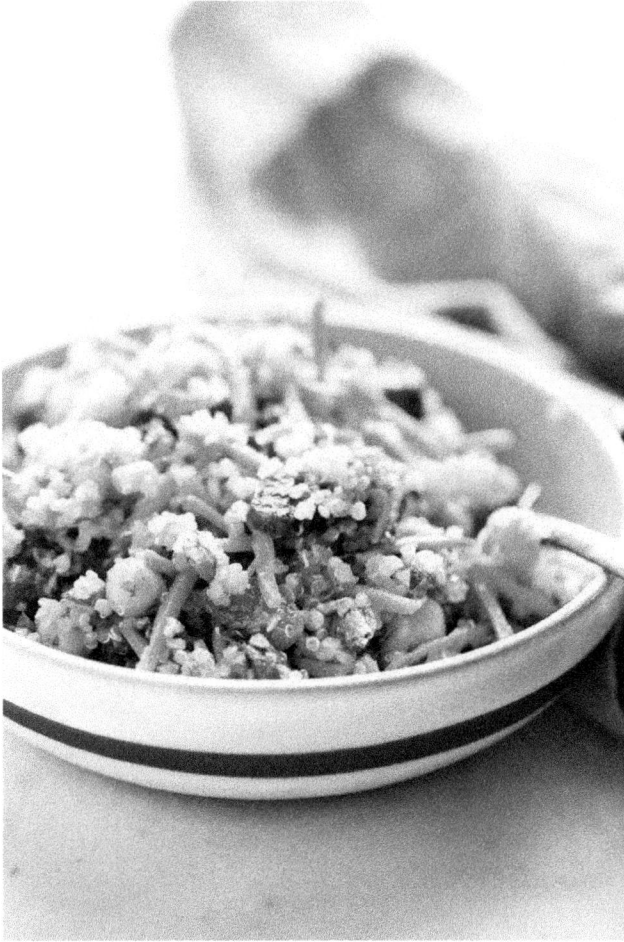

Ingredients:

- 1 can chickpeas, drained
- ½ cup chopped parsley
- cup cherry tomatoes, quartered
- 4 oz. feta cheese, cubed

- ½ cup red grapes, halved
- Salt and pepper to taste
- ¼ cup Greek yogurt
- tablespoons extra virgin olive oil 1 tablespoon lemon juice

Directions:

1.   Combine the chickpeas, parsley, tomatoes, grapes and feta cheese in a salad bowl.

2.   Add the rest of the ingredients and season with salt and pepper.

3.   Serve the salad as fresh as possible.

Creamy Cucumber Salad
Servings: 4

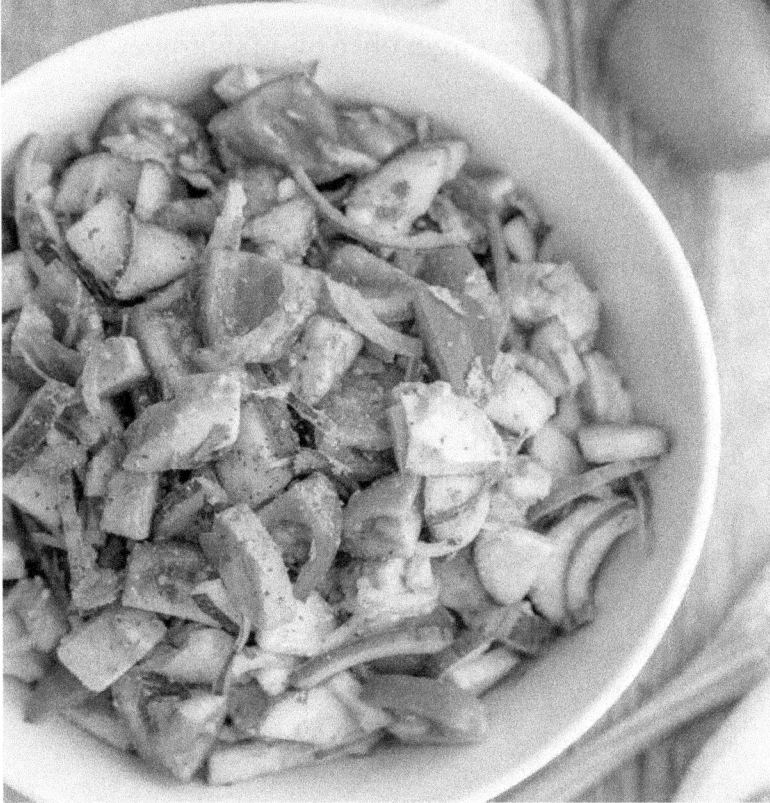

Ingredients:

- 4 cucumbers, diced
- 2 garlic cloves, minced
- 2 tablespoons chopped dill
- 1 teaspoon lemon juice
- ½ cup Greek yogurt Salt and pepper to taste

Directions:

1.   Combine the cucumbers and the rest of the ingredients in a salad bowl.

2.   Season with salt and pepper and serve the salad fresh.

Grilled Salmon Bulgur Salad
Servings: 4

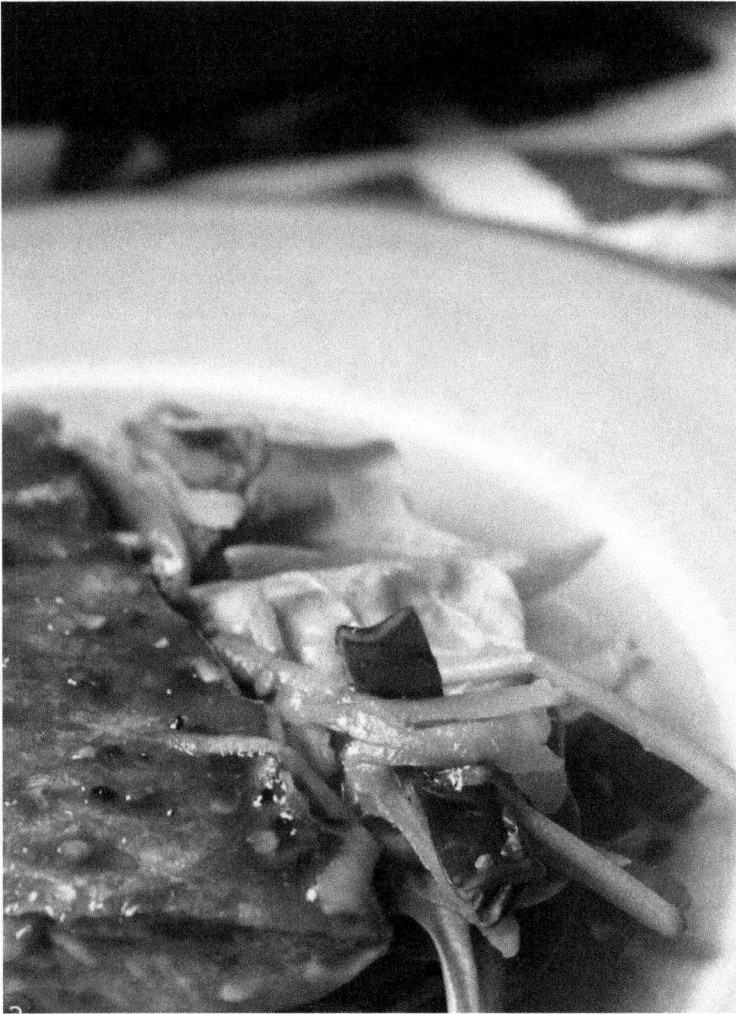

Ingredients:

- 2 salmon fillets
- Salt and pepper to taste
- ½ cup bulgur
- 2 cups vegetable stock

- 1 cup cherry tomatoes, halved 1 cucumber, cubed
- 1 green onion, chopped
- ½ cup green olives, sliced
- 1 red bell pepper, cored and diced
- 1 red pepper, chopped
- ½ cup sweet corn 1 lemon, juiced

Directions:

1. Season the salmon with salt and pepper and place it on a hot grill pan. Cook it on each side until browned.

2. Combine the bulgur and stock in a saucepan. Cook until all the liquid has been absorbed then transfer in a salad bowl.

3. Add the rest of the ingredients, including the salmon and season with salt and pepper.

4. Serve the salad fresh.

Roasted Bell Pepper Arugula Salad
Servings: 4

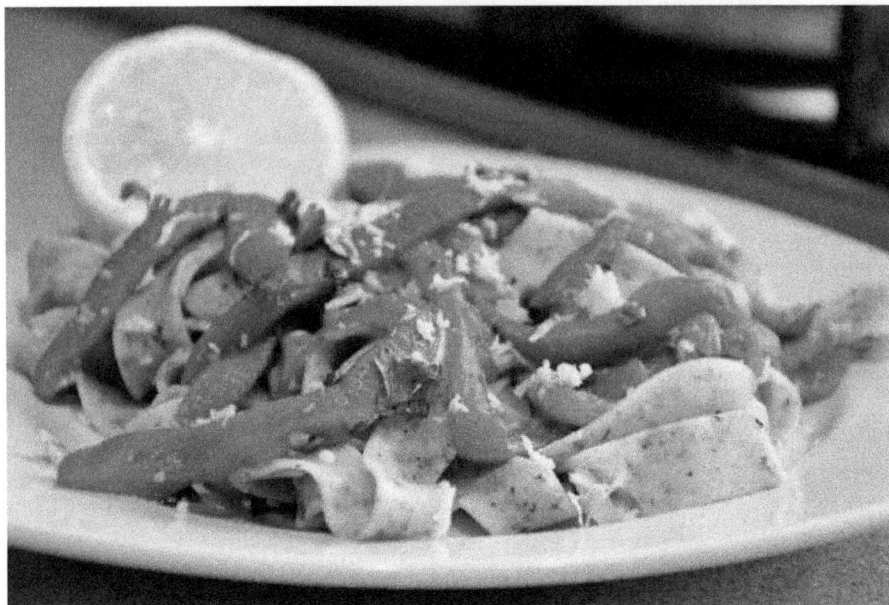

Ingredients

- 3   cups arugula
- 6 roasted red bell peppers, sliced 1 red onion, sliced
- 4 oz. feta cheese, crumbled 2 tablespoons dried raisins
- 2 tablespoons pine nuts Salt and pepper to taste
- 2 tablespoons balsamic vinegar
- 2 tablespoons extra virgin olive oil

Directions:

1.   Combine the bell peppers, red onion, raisins, pine nuts, vinegar and oil in a bowl.

2.   Add the arugula and mix gently then top with feta cheese and serve the salad fresh.

Garlicky Roasted Bell Pepper Salad
Servings: 4

Ingredients:

- 8 roasted red bell peppers, sliced
- 1 cup cherry tomatoes, halved
- 2 tablespoons chopped parsley
- 4 garlic cloves, minced
- 1 shallot, sliced
- 2 tablespoons extra virgin olive oil
- 1 tablespoon balsamic vinegar
- pinch chili flakes
- tablespoons pine nuts
- Salt and pepper to taste

Directions

1. Combine all the ingredients in a salad bowl.

2. Add salt and pepper and mix well.

3. Serve the salad as fresh as possible.

Roasted Vegetable Salad
Servings: 6

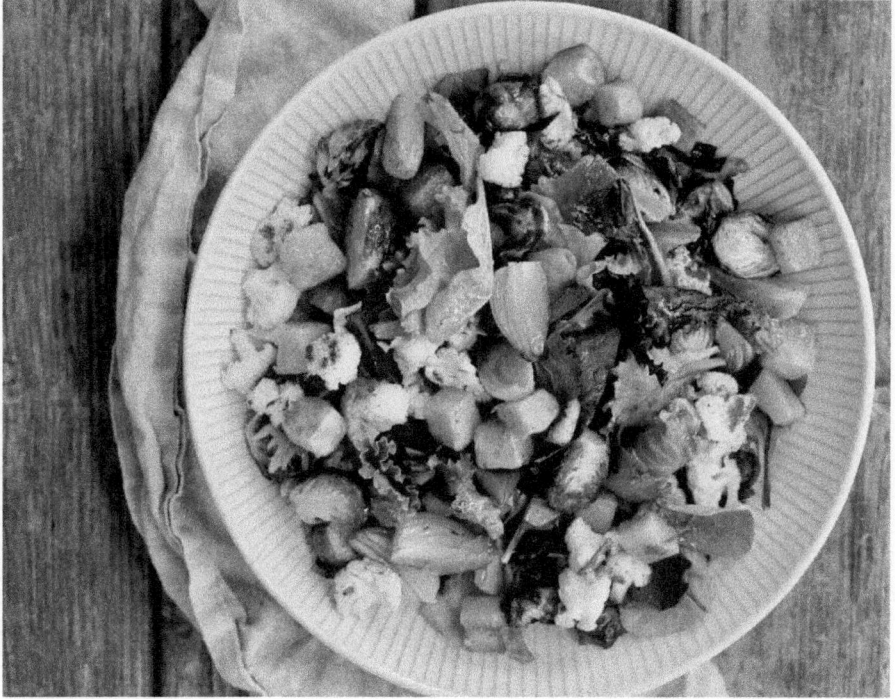

Ingredients:

- ½ pound baby carrots
- 2 red onions, sliced
- zucchini, sliced
- eggplants, cubed
- 1 cauliflower, cut into florets
- 1 sweet potato, peeled and cubed 1 endive, sliced
- tablespoons extra virgin olive oil 1 teaspoon dried basil
- Salt and pepper to taste 1 lemon, juiced
- 1 tablespoon balsamic vinegar

Directions:

1.   Combine the vegetables with the oil, basil, salt and pepper in a deep dish baking pan and cook in the preheated oven at 350F for 25-30 minutes.

2.   When done, transfer in a salad bowl and add the lemon juice and vinegar.

3.   Serve the salad fresh.

Chickpea Arugula Salad
Servings: 4

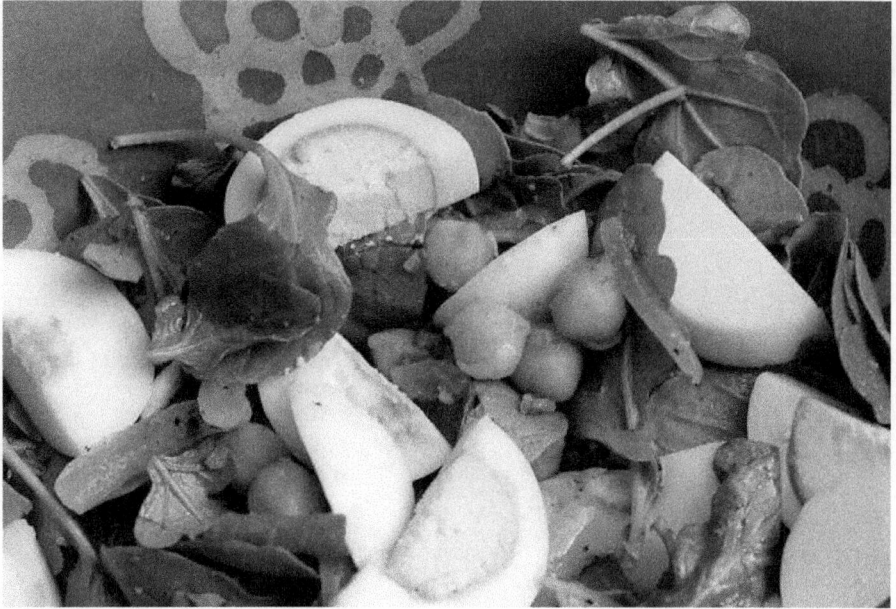

Ingredients:

- 1 can chickpeas, drained
- 1 cup cherry tomatoes, halved
- 1/2cup sun-dried tomatoes, chopped 2 cups arugula
- 1 pita bread, cubed
- ½ cup black olives, pitted
- 1 shallot, sliced
- ½ teaspoon cumin seeds
- ½ teaspoon coriander seeds
- ¼ teaspoon chili powder
- 1 teaspoon chopped mint Salt and pepper to taste
- 4 oz. goat cheese, crumbled

Directions:

1.   Combine the chickpeas, tomatoes, arugula, pita bread, olives, shallot, spices and mint in a salad bowl.

2.   Add salt and pepper to taste and mix well then stir in the cheese.

3.   Serve the salad fresh.

Greek Chicken Salad
Servings: 2

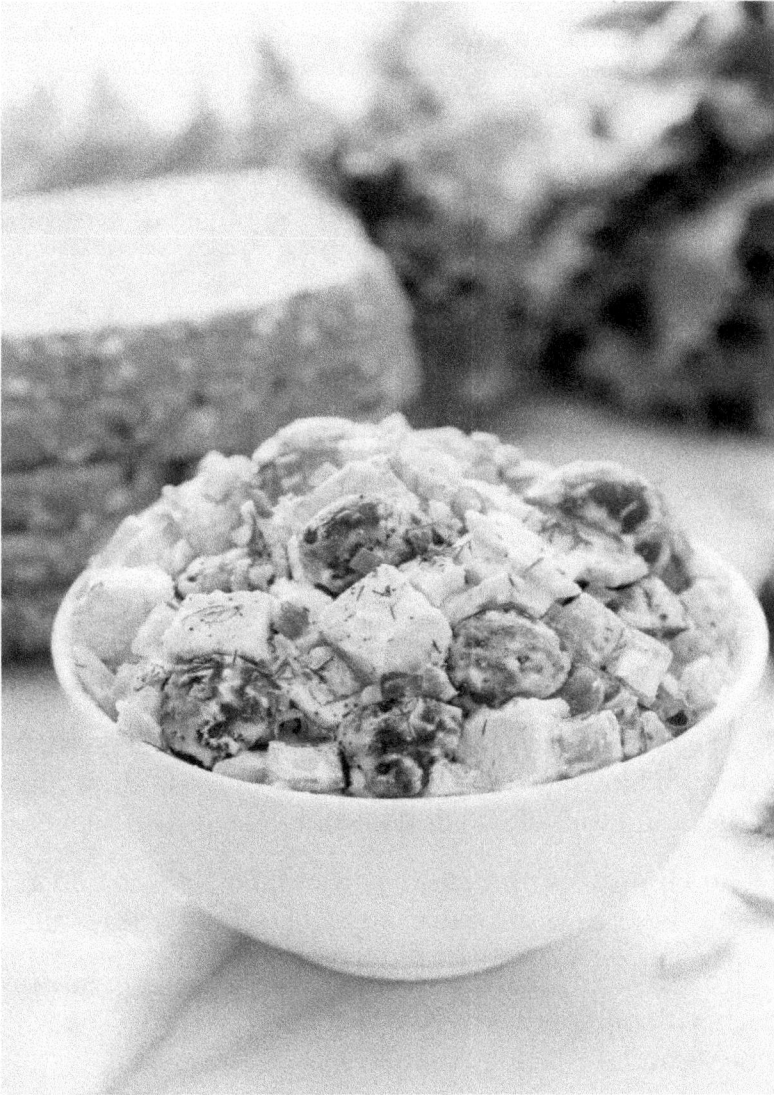

Ingredients

- 1/4 cup balsamic vinegar

- 1/2 cup thinly sliced red onion

- 1 teaspoon freshly squeezed lemon juice

- 1/4 cup extra-virgin olive oil

- 1/4 teaspoon salt

- 1/4 teaspoon freshly ground black pepper

- 2 grilled boneless, skinless chicken breasts, sliced (about 1 cup)

- 10 cherry tomatoes, halved

- 8 pitted Kalamata olives, halved

- 2 cups roughly chopped romaine lettuce

- 1/2 cup feta cheese

Directions

1. In a medium bowl, combine the vinegar and lemon juice and stir well. Slowly whisk in the olive oil and continue whisking vigorously until well blended. Whisk in the salt and pepper.

2. Add the olives, tomatoes, onions, and chicken and stir well. for at least 2 hours or overnight, Cover and refrigerate.

3. To serve, divide the romaine between 2 salad plates and top each with half of the chicken vegetable mixture. Top with feta cheese and serve immediately.

Greek-Style Picnic Salad

Servings: 10

Ingredients:

- 2 cups of Uncooked White Rice
- 3/4 cups of Sun-Dried Tomatoes
- 8 cups of Spinach
- 1 1/2 tablespoons of Olive Oil
- 1 cup of Boiling Water
- 2 cloves of Minced Garlic
- 2 cups of Crumbled Reduced-Fat Feta Cheese
- 1 teaspoon of Dried Oregano
- 1/4 cup of Chopped Pitted Kalamata Olives
- 1/2 teaspoon of Ground Black Pepper
- 1/2 teaspoon of Salt
- 15 1/2 ounces of Chickpeas
- 3 tablespoons of Toasted Pine Nuts
- 10 Lemon Wedges

Directions:

1.   Cook your rice according to the package instructions. Omit fat and salt. Cool to the room temperature and set aside.

2.   Combine your boiling water and sun-dried tomatoes in a bowl. Let stand for approximately 30 minutes until tomatoes are soft. Drain and cut tomatoes into 1-inch pieces.

3.   Heat 1 1/2 teaspoons of oil in a skillet over a medium-high heat. Add your garlic and spinach. Saute for 3 minutes until the spinach wilts. Combine your tomatoes, rice, cheese, spinach mixture, chickpeas, salt, pepper, olives, oregano, and feta cheese. Drizzle with your 1 remaining tablespoon of oil. Toss it together gently to coat. Sprinkle your pine nuts on top and add your lemon wedges to the side.

4.   Serve and Enjoy!

Mediterranean Detox Salad

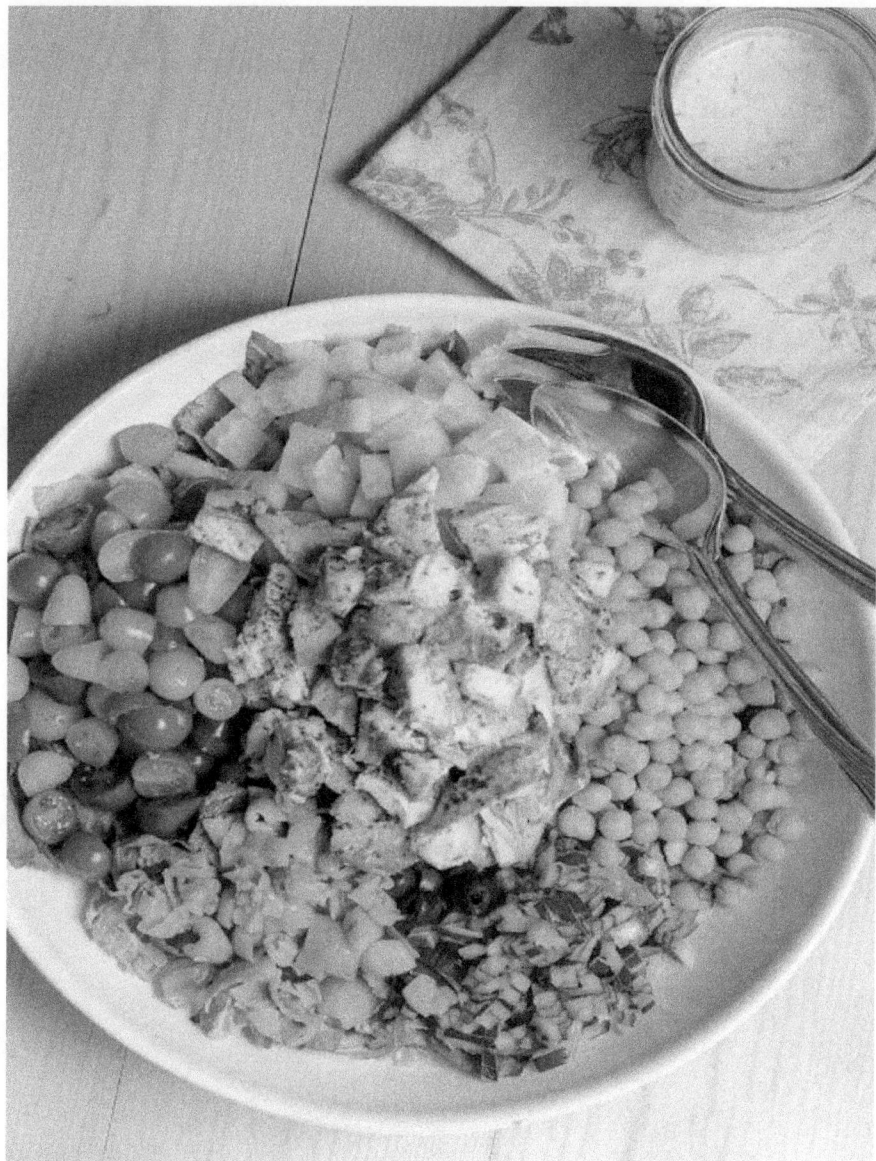

Ingredients:

*   8-ounce English Cucumber

- 2 tablespoons of Extra-Virgin Olive Oil

- 2 tablespoons of Fresh Lemon Juice

- 6 cups of Trimmed Watercress

- 1/2 cup of Feta Cheese

- 1/2 cup of Sliced Red Onion

- 2 Large Celery Stalks

- 14-ounce can of Artichoke Hearts (quartered)

- Black Pepper

Directions:

1.   Cut your cucumber in half and then slice it crosswise into 1/4- inch thick slices. Add a 3/4 cup of your cucumber and lemon juice to your blender and process. Add olive oil and pulse until it is all combined. Season your dressing with black pepper. Transfer to a large bowl.

2.   Add your remaining 1 cup of cucumber, artichoke hearts, watercress, red onion, feta cheese, and celery to a bowl. Toss it with your dressing.

3.   Divide salad equally among 4 bowls.

4.   Serve and Enjoy!

Two-Bean Greek Salad

Servings: 4

Ingredients:

- 3/4 pound of String Beans

- 2 teaspoons of Dijon Mustard

- 2 tablespoons of Red Wine Vinegar

- 4 1/2 teaspoons of Olive Oil

- 3 teaspoons of Chopped Fresh Oregano

- 1/2 teaspoon of Ground Black Pepper

- 10 ounces of Shelled Frozen Edamame

- 1 cup of Grape Tomatoes

- 3 ounces of Haloumi Cheese (Sliced Into 4 Pieces)

- 1/4 cup of Pitted Kalamata Olives

- 2 Multi-Grain Pitas

Directions:

1.   In your bowl, whisk together red wine vinegar, 2 teaspoons of olive oil, 2 1/2 teaspoons of oregano, and 1/4 teaspoon of pepper. Set to the side.

2.   Place your steamer basket in your saucepan filled with a couple inches of water. Cook your edamame while covered. Should take about 3 minutes until tender. Transfer to a bowl. Add your string beans to the steamer and cook while covered for about 2 minutes. Add your beans to the edamame. Add your olives and tomatoes. Toss it all to combine.

3.   Heat your oiled grill pan over a medium-high heat. Brush a tablespoon of oil on one side of your pitas. Turn it until golden.

Should take 2 minutes to cook. Transfer your pitas to your plate. Brush 1/2 teaspoon of your oil evenly on one side of your cheese slices. Sprinkle your remaining pepper and oregano on them. Grill the cheese with the seasoned side down, until you see marks begin to form. Should take approximately 1 minute. Transfer to your plate.

4.   Place a pita half on each of your 4 plates. Top them with your bean salad and cheese. Drizzle the remaining olive oil on top.

5.   Serve and Enjoy!

Mediterranean Brown Rice Salad

Servings: 6

Ingredients:

- 1 Thinly Sliced Red Bell Pepper

- 1 1/2 cups of Uncooked Brown Rice

- 3 cups of Water

- 1/4 cup of Feta Cheese

- 1 cup of Thawed Frozen Green Peas

- 1/4 Chopped Sweet Onion

- 1/2 cup of Raisins

- 1/4 cup of Chopped Kalamata Olives

- 1/4 cup of Balsamic Vinegar

- 1/2 cup of Vegetable Oil

- 1 1/4 teaspoons of Dijon Mustard

- Salt

- Ground Black Pepper

Directions:

1.   Bring your brown rice and water to a boil over a high heat in your saucepan. Reduce the heat to a medium-low. Cover and simmer until your rice has become tender and all the liquid is absorbed. Should take approximately 45 to 50 minutes.

2.   Combine your peas, onion, raisins, bell pepper, and olives in a big bowl.

3. Whisk your vinegar, vegetable oil, and mustard together in a different bowl for your balsamic dressing.

4. Stir your brown rice and balsamic dressing into your vegetable mix. Season with black pepper and salt.

5. Top your brown rice and vegetables with your feta cheese.

6. Serve and Enjoy!

Heirloom Tomato Salad with Pearl Couscous

Servings: 10

Ingredients:

- 1 cup of Pearl Couscous
- 2 cups of Vegetable Stock
- 1/2 cup of Fresh Basil Leaves
- 1/2 cup + 1 tablespoon of Extra-Virgin Olive Oil
- 1/4 cup of Flat-Leaf Parsley Leaves
- 1 clove of Crushed Garlic
- 1 tablespoon of Chopped Fresh Thyme
- 1 tablespoon of Chopped Fresh Oregano
- 1/2 cup of Pitted Green Olives
- 15 Cherry Tomatoes (Quartered)
- 4 Heirloom Tomatoes (Quartered)
- 1 Cubed English Cucumber
- 1 cup of Crumbled Feta Cheese
- 1/2 Small Thinly Sliced Red Onion
- 1/4 cup of White Balsamic Vinegar
- 1 Juiced Lemon

Directions:

1.   Bring your vegetable stock to a simmer over a medium heat in your saucepan. Heat 1 tablespoon of olive oil in your skillet over a medium heat. Stir in your couscous and cook until

it is golden brown. Stir occasionally. Should take about 10 minutes.

2.   Stir your toasted couscous into your hot vegetable stock and return it to a simmer. Cover and cook until your stock has been absorbed into your couscous. Should take about 15 minutes. Scrape into your mixing bowl, fluff it using your fork and allow to cool until it reaches room temperature.

3.   Place your garlic, basil, oregano, parsley, olives, and thyme into your food processor. Pulse until all your herbs are chopped coarsely. Stir your herb mixture into your couscous along with your cherry tomatoes, heirloom tomatoes, red onion, feta cheese, and cucumber. Drizzle with your lemon juice, 1/2 cup of olive oil, and vinegar. Stir it all together until it is evenly combined.

4.   Serve and Enjoy!

Kashi, Mint, and Almond Salad

Servings: 4

Ingredients:

- 1 Small Chopped Onion
- 4 tablespoons of Extra-Virgin Olive Oil
- 2 cloves of Minced Garlic
- 2 teaspoons of Ground Cumin
- 1 cup of Uncooked Kashi 7 Whole Grain Pilaf
- 3 tablespoons of Fresh Lemon Juice
- 2 Bay Leaves
- 5 tablespoons of Sliced Natural Almonds
- 1/4 cup of Chopped Parsley
- 1/4 cup of Chopped Fresh Mint
- 8 Cherry Tomatoes
- 4 Large Romaine Leaves
- Coarse Salt
- Ground Black Pepper

Directions:

1.   In a large sized saucepan, heat up 2 tablespoons of oil over a medium heat. Add your onion and season with pepper and salt. Cook onion until tender and browned lightly. Stir it occasionally. Should take about 5 minutes. Add garlic and cumin. Cook until fragrant. Should take approximately 1 minute.

2.   Add your Kashi, bay leaves, pepper, salt, and 2 cups of water. Bring to a boil. Reduce your heat to a simmer, cover, and continue to cook until your Kashi is tender. Should take approximately 40 minutes. Transfer to your bowl. Remove and get rid of the bay leaves. Add your lemon juice and the remaining oil. Allow to cool to room temperature for 20 minutes.

3.   Add tomatoes, mint, parsley, and 4 tablespoons of almonds. Toss well.

4.   Place a romaine leaf on 4 different plates. Spoon your mixture onto the center of your leaves. Drizzle with oil and sprinkle your remaining almonds on top.

5.   Serve and Enjoy!

Bean Salad w/ Balsamic Vinaigrette

Servings: 6

Ingredients:

- Vinaigrette:
- 2 tablespoons of Balsamic Vinegar
- 4 Finely Chopped Garlic Cloves
- 1/3 cup of Chopped Fresh Parsley
- 1/4 cup of Extra-Virgin Olive Oil
- 15 ounce can of Garbanzo Beans
- 15 ounce can of Black Beans
- 1 Medium Diced Red Onion
- 1/2 cup of Finely Chopped Celery
- 6 Lettuce Leaves
- Ground Black Pepper

Directions:

1. For your vinaigrette, whisk together your parsley, balsamic vinegar, pepper, and garlic in a small bowl. While your whisking, slowly add your olive oil. Set off to the side.

2. In a big bowl, combine your onion and beans. Pour your vinaigrette over your mixture and gently toss to mix it well and coat evenly. Cover your bowl and refrigerate.

3.   Place one lettuce leaf on each of your 6 plates. Divide your salad among these plates and garnish with your chopped celery.

4.   Serve and Enjoy!

Mediterranean Tuna Antipasto Salad

Servings: 4

Ingredients:

•   19-ounce can of Chickpeas

•   2 6-ounce cans of Water Packed Light Tuna (Drained & Flaked)

•   1/2 cup of Finely Chopped Red Onion

•   1 Large Finely Diced Red Bell Pepper

•   4 teaspoons of Capers

•   1/2 cup of Chopped Fresh Parsley

•   1/2 cup of Lemon Juice

•   1 1/2 teaspoons of Finely Chopped Fresh Rosemary

•   4 tablespoons of Extra-Virgin Olive Oil

•   8 cups of Mixed Salad Greens

•   1/4 teaspoon of Salt

•   Ground Pepper

Directions:

1.   Combine your tuna, beans, onion, pepper, capers, parsley, rosemary, 1/4 cup of lemon juice, and 2 tablespoons of oil in a medium bowl. Season with pepper.

2.   Combine your remaining 1/4 cup of lemon juice, salt, and 2 tablespoons of oil in a large bowl. Add your salad greens and

toss to coat. Divide your greens on to 4 plates. Top each of them with your tuna salad.

3.   Serve and Enjoy!

Walnut & Beet Salad

Servings: 4

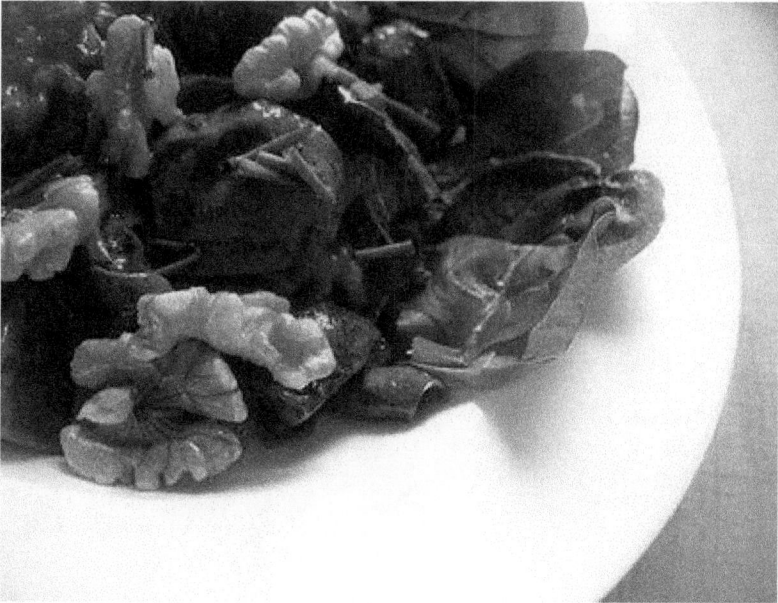

Ingredients:

- 3 cups of Beets

- 1/4 cup of Red Wine Vinegar

- 1 tablespoon of Water

- 1 tablespoon of Olive Oil

- 3 tablespoons of Balsamic Vinegar

- 1/4 cup of Chopped Apple

- 1/4 cup of Chopped Celery

- 8 cups of Fresh Salad Greens

- 3 tablespoons of Chopped Walnuts

- 1/4 cup of Crumbled Gorgonzola Cheese

- Ground Pepper

Directions:

1.   Steam your raw beets in water in a saucepan until they are tender. Slip off their skins. Rinse them to cool. Slice into 1/2-inch rounds.

2.   In a medium sized bowl, toss beets with red wine vinegar.

3.   In a big bowl, combine your olive oil, balsamic vinegar, and water. Add your salad greens and toss to combine.

4.   Put your greens onto individual plates. Top with your sliced beets, celery, and chopped apples. Sprinkle with your walnuts, pepper, and cheese.

5.   Serve and Enjoy!

Bean Salad & Toasted Pita

Servings: 4

Ingredients:

- 2 cups of Cooked Pinto Beans
- 2 tablespoons of Fresh Lemon Juice
- 1 1/2 teaspoons of Salt
- 3 cloves of Peeled Garlic
- 2 tablespoons of Toasted Cumin Seeds
- 1 cup of Diced Plum Tomatoes
- 5 tablespoons of Extra-Virgin Olive Oil
- 1/2 cup of Sliced Romaine Lettuce
- 1/2 Peeled and Diced Cucumber
- 1 cup of Crumbled Feta Cheese
- 3 tablespoons of Chopped Fresh Mint
- 3 tablespoons of Chopped Fresh Parsley
- 1 Small Chopped Onion
- Whole Wheat Pita Breads (Cut Into Bite Sized Pieces)
- Ground Pepper

Directions:

1. Place your beans in a large bowl, cover with 3-inches of cold water and allow to soak for at least 4 hours.

2. Heat olive oil in a large saucepan over a medium heat. Add onion and 1 clove of garlic. Cook for 3 to 4 minutes until

mixture begin to soften. Drain your beans and add to your pan. Add enough water to cover the beans by an inch. Boil for 5 minutes. Lower the heat to a simmer, partially cover your pan and cook for 20 minutes to 3 hours until tender. Time will depend on the freshness of the beans being used. If the water drops below the beans at any time, add in an additional cup of hot water.

3.   Preheat your oven to 400 degrees. Spread the pita pieces out on a baking sheet. Bake for 5 to 7 minutes until crisp. Allow to cool on your pan.

4.   Mash 2 cloves of garlic and 1/2 teaspoon of salt with the back of your knife to form a paste. Move to a bowl. Add your cumin and lemon juice. Whisk to blend it all together. Add in 2 tablespoons of olive oil whisking continually. Season this dressing with your pepper.

5.   Place your beans, cucumber, and tomatoes in serving bowl. Add your toasted pita, feta, lettuce, parsley, mint, and the dressing. Toss it all together until mixed. Season with more pepper.

6.   Serve and Enjoy!

CPSIA information can be obtained
at www.ICGtesting.com
Printed in the USA
BVHW041508180321
602887BV00012B/1787

9 781801 454827